ADOLESCENT PSYCHIATRY
A Practical Guide

Dorothy Stubbe, M.D.
Associate Professor of Child Psychiatry
Training Director, Child and Adolescent Psychiatry
Yale Child Study Center
New Haven, Connecticut

. Lippincott Williams & Wilkins
a Wolters Kluwer business
Philadelphia · Baltimore · New York · London
Buenos Aires · Hong Kong · Sydney · Tokyo

Acquisitions Editor/Publisher: Charles W. Mitchell
Senior Managing Editor: Lisa R. Kairis
Project Manager: Fran Gunning
Manufacturing Manager: Ben Rivera
Associate Director of Marketing: Adam Glazer
Creative Director: Doug Smock
Production Services: International Typesetting and Composition
Printer: R.R. Donnelley, Crawfordsville

Library of Congress Cataloging-in-Publication Data

Stubbe, Dorothy.
    Child & adolescent psychiatry : a practical guide / Dorothy Stubbe.
        p. ; cm.
    Includes bibliographical references and index.
    ISBN-13: 978-0-7817-7831-2 (alk. paper)
    ISBN-10: 0-7817-7831-X (alk. paper)
    1. Child psychiatry—Case studies.   2. Adolescent psychiatry—Case studies.
I. Title.   II. Title: Child and adolescent psychiatry.
    [DNLM: 1. Mental Disorders—diagnosis—Case Reports.   2. Adolescent.
3. Child.   4. Infant.   5. Mental Disorders—therapy—Case Reports. WS 350
S9324c 2007]
RJ499.S78 2007
618.92'89—dc22

                                                                2006018687

This book is dedicated to the sources of my inspiration: my wonderful family (John, Grace, and Caleb), my residents and students, and the children and families who have entrusted themselves to my care.

Preface

Working with troubled children and families is invigorating, rewarding, fascinating, frustrating, and confusing. Child and adolescent psychiatry is a discipline that can seem overwhelming at first. There are parents, schools, protective services, primary care physicians and many others providers with whom to collaborate. There are the complexities of the diagnostic interview with a child, which may require an enormous amount of creativity to help this child feel comfortable enough to engage, let alone communicate to you the personal information required for psychiatric understanding. It is a field that pulls at your most basic emotions—such as the wish to "adopt" your patients, over-identification with the vulnerability of the child patient, and wanting to undo the actions of "incompetent" parents. We are mandated reporters, which may necessitate "turning in" parents to authorities. We are the professional experts called on by schools, courts, and social service agencies to make decisions that have a profound effect on the child and family, including decisions about hospitalization, custody, placement, and even incarceration. We undertake the intense work of supporting dying children and grieving parents. We are called on to answer complex developmental and behavioral questions from parents, pediatricians, other professionals, and the media. These are the tasks of learning the art and science of child and adolescent psychiatry.

I vividly recall a child interview during my residency. I was called to the emergency department to evaluate a 10-year-old child who had been referred by the school because she had threatened to kill her teacher. My job, as delineated in a short memo from the school principal, was to attest to her safety, determine if the legal system or mental health system should be involved, and plan for her ongoing education if I was unable to ensure that she would be completely safe at school. So, shouldering that heavy burden, I entered the room to investigate these matters. There, sitting sullenly, was a 10-(appearing 16-) year-old African American girl who was with an emergency department "sitter" (the school had sent her alone by ambulance, and her mother was at work and couldn't take off or she would lose her job, according to the social worker who had done an initial intake history). I introduced myself and began to launch into the history and mental status exam when, in sudden realization, I stopped short. The girl was not answering my questions. She had turned her back on me and was totally and utterly silent. Was she psychotic, angry, oppositional, dissociating? I asked "are you hearing voices?" to which I received a curt reply—"No, you f—ing moron. Just get out of here!" Actually, that was a tempting proposition at that point, but I had my job to do. I sat a good long while thinking. Finally, I reached over for some play doh (which was there for monitored play) and began to squish at it and offered her some, which she finally picked up and squished as well. Finally, at my wit's end, I said the obvious. "Well, what to do? I guess you don't want to be here and you are stuck with a psychiatrist who is supposed to figure out if you are safe. What do *you* suggest we do?" She gazed at me for the first time, looking incredulous. "What do you mean, what do *I* suggest? You are the shrink! You can read my mind. You tell me!" I admitted that, actually, I could not read her mind (I wasn't completely sure that she knew that) and that I did not know what to do—but I *would* like to hear her side of the story of what happened at school. To my utter amazement, *she told me*. She told of living in a scary neighborhood where only the tough survive—and she was a survivor. She told me she was not very smart (which was actually not at all true) and of the indignities foisted on her by her teacher when she did not know an answer. "I guess I just couldn't take it anymore," was her final statement.

The girl was admitted to the children's psychiatric inpatient unit, where I was rotating. I was her doctor. I learned many things from her (and from the fabulous supervision I received around her care). I learned that children are not just miniature adults even though (as in her case) they may look like it. I learned that engaging with a child uses many modalities. I learned that what is asked by schools and others may be impossible to do or, even more importantly, may not even be the right questions to ask. I learned that children know honesty when they see it—and they know when they are being manipulated. I learned that building rapport with both the child or adolescent and his or her caregiver (either one alone will not do) is the essence of any treatment. I learned that there are no books to address the must-know practicalities of child and adolescent psychiatric care. I could learn the Diagnostic and Statistical Manual (DSM). I could learn about psychopharmacology, epidemiology, and components of a workup. But I longed for a practical "how to" guide that would provide helpful advice in my work with complicated patients, situations, and dilemmas.

The Practical Guide series is just that—a series of manuals that provide practical, user friendly, and engaging material that may be used in clinical practice. I chose to write this manual on child and adolescent psychiatry because, as a former trainee, as a clinician educator, and now as a training director for child and adolescent psychiatry residents, these are the gems that I have accumulated. This is the advice I now attempt to impart to residents. This manual serves as an organization of the pearls of clinical practice in child and adolescent psychiatry—from mnemonics to recall diagnostic criteria to clinical vignettes to important tips for working with children and systems. This is a manual that may be used by child and adolescent psychiatry residents and many more— medical students, psychiatry residents, other mental health professionals, and even more seasoned practitioners.

Working with children and families with psychiatric disabilities is, in my mind, the most fascinating, needed, and rewarding of all careers. I hope this manual conveys my love and dedication to children, to my profession, and to teaching. This manual does not take the place of textbooks, journals, literature reviews, intensive supervision, or clinical experience. However, I do hope that this book will find its way into the pockets of and be useful to all clinicians who embark on the crucial mission of treating children who are suffering from psychiatric disorders.

Contents

I

GENERAL PRINCIPLES OF DEVELOPMENT AND THE PSYCHIATRIC EVALUATION OF CHILDREN AND ADOLESCENTS

1 ▼ Overview of Development

Essential Concepts
- Children are not just miniature adults.
- Child development entails a complex inter-action between genetic potential, biological capacities, and the nurturing environment.
- Assessment of developmental strengths (competencies), as well as psychopathology (areas of need), is essential to a complete psychiatric assessment of the child, adolescent, and his/her family.

Whoever touches the life of the child touches the most sensitive point of a whole which has roots in the most distant past and climbs toward the infinite future.

—Maria Montessori

DEVELOPMENTAL STAGES

What development is *not* is consistent and unalterable. The normal range of development is broad, and one stage does not neatly finish before the next can begin. However, recalling these stages is much more useful than merely studying for Board examinations. It keeps in mind the need to think developmentally, to consider the areas of development in which a child is doing well, and the areas in which he or she needs intervention. Although seeing hundreds of children (both typical and impaired) is the best way to begin to differentiate normal variations in temperament and fantasy from more concerning symptoms of psychiatric disorder, the tried and true developmental models, particularly that of Erikson, may be useful for the ongoing assessment of a child's ability to meet and master the developmental tasks at each age. Each time I assess a child or adolescent, I review in my own mind the developmental tasks for the age, and how the child is faring with respect to these. For children and adolescents, treatment is not merely focused on a specific diagnostic disorder, but on providing interventions that address areas of developmental concern, and helping the child gain the skills and support needed to get on a healthier developmental trajectory.

A basic understanding of human development is fundamental to the psychiatric evaluation in general and most essential in the assessment of children and adolescents. An appreciation for the wide variability among children in terms of development will assist in identifying and targeting areas of developmental concern while minimizing the risk of over-diagnosis and overpathologizing. Normal reactions of one developmental period (such as stranger anxiety in a 1-year-old) when it occurs in another stage (such as similar severe fears in a 5-year-old) may suggest a disorder.

✛ KEY POINT

I would like to emphasize at the very beginning of the book what I consider to be a key aspect of all of child and adolescent psychiatry which is frequently given short shrift. A thorough evaluation and treatment plan for a child, adolescent, or family needs to highlight areas of *strength and resilience*, not merely pathology. In child and adolescent psychiatry, many of the children we see have suffered severe psychosocial adversity, family chaos, abuse or neglect, have unsafe behaviors, and meet DSM-IV criteria for multiple disorders. In this context, sorting out the risk factors and pathology may dominate the therapeutic encounter. However, it is the assessment and appreciation of strengths that may most meaningfully build a therapeutic alliance, may provide our most accurate prognostic indicators, and may be the most useful method of choosing appropriate treatment modalities. I have found in each child or adolescent I assess or treat a unique inner "spark"—that part of her or him that is the healthiest, has the most hope, and is most amenable to treatment. Finding that "spark" within the patient may provide *insights far beyond those gleaned from diagnosing the disorder.*

Child and adolescent psychiatrists are, typically, first adult psychiatrists. It is thus easy to assume that children are just "miniature adults." A frequent error is in the supposition that our evaluations, diagnoses, and treatment plans can merely be "downsized" for the child or adolescent. In fact, the chronological unfolding of progressive capabilities and processes from infancy onward must be appreciated to understand and treat the patient as a whole. Treatments are different for individuals at different stages of development.

Theories of development have encompassed entire textbooks, so I will distill out the concepts that I believe are most essential in assessing children and adolescents who are referred for emotional or behavioral difficulties. The primary developmental theorists discussed will be Sigmund Freud (psychosexual stages), Erik Erikson (psychosocial stages), and Jean Piaget (cognitive stages). Additionally, some highlights of each of the developmental periods of childhood and adolescence will be mentioned, as well as risk factors for each stage. Table 1.1 compares the three developmental theorists.

PRENATAL DEVELOPMENT

Each person has 23 double helix strands of the genetic code for all physical characteristics and organ capacities in the body. Traits such as temperament and activity level also have a genetic basis. Although some genes have strong penetrance and express themselves in virtually all environments (such as eye color), much of development is the product of complex gene-environment interactions. Family history of development may give an indication of the genetic makeup and potential vulnerabilities of the fetus. Understanding the nurturing environment assists in gaining an appreciation for the unfolding of the genetic potential in a given individual.

The second trimester of gestation is when neurological and brain development occurs most rapidly. Thus, insults during this time may result in obvious or more subtle functional deficits for the baby. The clinician should inquire about the prenatal period. Exposure to substances (alcohol, substances of abuse, or medications), trauma, or severe stress during pregnancy may be significant to the developing fetus and be a source of vulnerability when the baby is born.

INFANCY (BIRTH TO 1 YEAR)

Sigmund Freud characterized infancy as the *Oral Stage* of development, during which time the mouth and eating were of dominant importance. This stage is marked by extreme dependency, urgency of needs, low frustration tolerance, and no consideration of others. Erik Erikson, in his psychosocial stages of development, postulated the normative crisis of infancy as

TABLE 1.1. Comparison of Developmental Theorists

Age	Sigmund Freud **Psychoanalytic drive theory** **Psychosexual stages**	Erik Erikson **Psychoanalytic theory** **Psychosocial stages**	Jean Piaget **Cognitive stages of development**
0–1	**Oral Stage** (birth to 12–18 mo) Primary site of gratification and tension in oral area (mouth, lips, tongue) Sucking and biting	**Trust vs. Mistrust** (birth to 12–18 mo) Trust depends on reliability of care provided by caretaker Frustration associated with weaning Optimism and hope derive from basic trust	**Sensorimotor Phase** (birth–2 yr) Modification of reflexes; cross modal fluency Association between means and ends Object permanence; objects still exist even if obscured from view Mastery motivation (10–12 mo); child seeks to master challenges
1–3	**Anal Phase** (12–18 to 36 mo) Primary site of tension and gratification is anal area Toilet training	**Autonomy vs. Shame** (12–18 to 36 mo) Increased capacities (motor, sphincter, language, etc.) Need for consistent limits from caretaker Shame occurs with lack of self-control Self-doubt evolves from parental shaming	Can infer cause and effect (1–2 yr) Schemas (units or categories of cognition) Assimilation (incorporation of new knowledge) and accommodation (modification of schema to adapt to new stimuli)

(Continued)

TABLE 1.1. Comparison of Developmental Theorists *(continued)*

Age	Sigmund Freud	Erik Erikson	Jean Piaget
3–5	**Phallic-Oedipal Phase** (3–5 yr) Primary site of tension and gratification—genitals Castration anxiety, fear of genital loss or injury (interest in Band-Aids) Oedipus complex: Child desires intimacy with parent of opposite sex; to be rid of same-sex parent	**Initiative vs. Guilt** (3–5 yr) Initiative, enjoyment of activity and accomplishments Guilt over aggressive urges Resolution of oedipal conflict via role identification Sibling rivalry common	**Preoperational Phase** (2–6 yr) Language acquisition and symbolic reasoning Egocentrism; see world exclusively from own perspective Thinking is transductive (causality inferred from temporal or spatial proximity) Magic thinking (prelogical)
6–11	**Latency Stage** (6–11 yr) Relative quiescence of libidinal drives Sexual drives channeled into socially appropriate activities (i.e., school work, sports) Further development of ego functions Formation of superego Focus on same-sex relationships	**Industry vs. inferiority** (6–11 yr) School is important Child is busy creating, building, accomplishing Danger of sense of inferiority and inadequacy of child; feels unable to compete with regard to skills (e.g., academic, sports) and status among peers Socially decisive age	**Concrete Operations** (6–11 yr) Emergence of logical, cause and effect thinking Reversibility of events and ideas Switch from egocentric to social speech Ability to see another's point of view Conservation of volume and quantity Rigid interpretation of rules

11 +	**Adolescent Genital Phase**	**Identity vs. Role Confusion**	**Formal Operations** (11 yr+)
	(11 or 12 yr and beyond)	(11–18 yr)	Hypothetical/deductive abstract reasoning
	Final stage of psychosexual development	Group identity (peers) primary	Elaboration of information processing
	Recapitulates earlier phases	Developing ego identity (sense of inner sameness)	Metacognitive capacity; can think about thinking
	Separation from family	Preoccupation with appearance	Ability to grasp concept of probabilities
	Identify formation	Moodiness and reactivity	
	Biological capacity for orgasm and psychological capacity for true intimacy develop	Danger of role confusion; uncertainty about sexual and vocational identity	

that *of Basic Trust vs. Mistrust.* The capacity for basic trust is achieved when the infant feels safe and well cared for by his or her caregivers. Infants gain a sense of security by having their physical needs cared for in a sensitive manner, according to John Bowlby. This caring and mutual bonding is the key to *secure attachment.*

Temperament is a person's inborn characteristic behavioral style. During infancy and the preschool years, temperament has moderate to high stability. Chess and Thomas have defined the dimensions of temperament. A temperamentally difficult child tends to demonstrate disrupted rhythmicity (irregularity of sleep cycles, feeding, and arousal states), social withdrawal, poor adaptability to change, intense emotional reactions, and negative mood. *Goodnesss of fit* describes a match between the parental expectations of the child and the child's temperament and innate capabilities. It is the mismatch that may predispose a child to (although not necessarily cause) behavioral or emotional problems. It is important to assess any mismatch between temperament and parental expectations, as early intervention may help reconcile the mismatch to improve developmental outcomes. All relationships entail interactions, and it is the reciprocal interactions between parent and child that determine the nature of the attachment process.

The infancy period is a time of rapid loss of cortical neurons, called *pruning.* An infant is born with a full complement of neurons, but they are not well interconnected. The pruning process allows for more specific interconnections to improve the efficiency of the nervous system—somewhat analogous to trying to get through a forest, which is slow and inefficient until a road is built by cutting down trees to make a well-organized path to the goal. Optimal stimulation (talking to the baby, looking at the baby, caring for the baby, and protecting the baby from extremes of neglect or chaos) can improve the efficiency of pruning, and thus assist in the developmental process. We now know that optimal stimulation during the early years of life is essential to optimal cortical efficiency. The brain is approximately one-third of its adult size at birth, and it grows rapidly, reaching 60% by approximately 1 year.

CLINICAL VIGNETTE

A mother brought her infant to the clinic due to failure to thrive. The 4-month-old infant (Thomas) was left buckled into his car seat on the other side of the room, awake but quiet. The mother sat down across from the intake clinician.

Interviewer:	*I notice Thomas is still in his car seat.*
Mother:	*Yes, that way we are able to talk.*
Interviewer:	*I notice that he is a little fussy. Perhaps you could hold him for a while?*
Mother:	*He'll be quiet soon [went over and put a pacifier in his mouth].*
Interviewer:	*It can be really demanding having an infant.*
Mother:	*You can say that again [looking completely depleted].*

The mother was quite depressed and emotionally unavailable to her child. This improved with her own treatment and regular meetings with in-home service professionals to help her *learn how to care for and interact with her child.*

Piaget characterized the infancy period as the Sensorimotor Stage, in which newborns demonstrate the ability to learn through making associations between means and ends. Beginning at about 6 months, object permanence evolves—the ability of a baby to know that an object does not cease to exist if it is out of sight. By the age of 1 to 2 years, the child can infer cause and effect. Schemas, or units or categories of cognition, organize memories. Thus, a dachshund is coded in the schema of "dog." Assimilation (incorporation of new knowledge) or accommodation (modification of schema to adapt to new stimuli) characterizes the coding of information for more efficient retrieval.

Dramatic changes in development that appear 2 to 3 months after birth are seen in both infants' behavior and the behavior of the caregiving adults. It is at about 2 months of age that the infant begins to smile at a face (*social smile*) and to imitate facial expressions of others. Parents are typically elated at this new capacity and may describe their child as "becoming a real person." The quantity of crying, which peaked at about 6 weeks, is beginning to diminish, and parents often report that, by this age, they are able to "read" (differentiate the cause of) their infant's cry. Even infants with colic (bouts of inconsolable crying totaling more than 3 hours daily for more than 3 days in any week in an infant that is otherwise healthy and well-fed) begin to calm, and colic usually disappears spontaneously by 4 months of age. Infants begin to babble at 3 to 4 months and to laugh by 4 months. At age 7 to 9 months, infants begin to act as if they understand that their thoughts, feelings, and actions can be communicated to, and understood by, another person, and they have strong preferences for caregivers with whom they have established relationships. Stranger anxiety, which peaks at about 8 to 9 months, emerges as the infant becomes increasingly attuned to comforting, familiar caregivers and becomes uncomfortable with unfamiliar people.

Risk factors in the infancy period include prematurity or serious illness in infancy, with increased risk for developmental difficulties and disruption of the parent–infant bonding process. However, even very premature infants frequently do well when the medical issues resolve. Other risk factors in the child are autism (a primary disorder of social relatedness), feeding problems (poor ability to suck and eat), and cognitive or overall developmental delay. Parental depression or other failures of attunement to the needs of the child (substance abuse, extreme stress, parental conflict, etc.) are also risk factors in the infancy period.

PRESCHOOL (2–5 YEARS)

Sigmund Freud's *Anal Stage* is said to be from age $1\frac{1}{2}$ to 3, and is thought to be associated with issues of control, orderliness, and cleanliness associated with toilet training. Erikson's psychosocial stage is that of *Autonomy vs. Shame,* in which a child may gain self-esteem through his or her increased capacities, whereas shame and self-doubt occur with lack of self-control and parental humiliations around toilet training. During Freud's *Phallic-Oedipal Phase* from 3 to 5 years, the primary site of tension and gratification is the genitals, and fear of injury, jealousy, and rivalry with the same-sexed parent are hallmarks. Erikson coined this the stage of conflicts between *Initiative and Guilt.* Initiative is the enjoyment of activity and accomplishment, whereas guilt is overaggressive urges that emerge at this stage. Role identification with the same-sexed parent is thought to occur at this time. This may also be known as the "Band-Aid" period, as even a miniscule injury requires the caring application of a Band-Aid.

Piaget's *Preoperational Stage* (ages 2–6) is characterized by explosive language development that ushers in the ability to reason symbolically rather than motorically, as in the sensorimotor period. The capacity for language development is genetically determined, but it is clearly enhanced by parental communication that is sensitive to the child's emerging abilities. Reasoning at this stage is transductive; that is, attribution of causality is based exclusively on temporal or spatial juxtaposition.

Judgments are dominated by immediate perceptions. Thinking is egocentric: the young child is conceptually unable to view events and experiences from any point of view but her own. Pretend play and fantasy thinking are common. This period is often characterized by imaginary friends and talking pets.

Risk factors for psychopathology at this age include severe behavior problems in the preschool period, which may predict multiple difficulties into adolescence. However, some defiant and aggressive behavior is normative in this age group, as children struggle to define themselves as unique individuals (sometimes referred to as the "terrible twos"). Developmental delays may become more obvious at this time, including language and motor difficulties, social difficulties, or the ability of a child to manage stress and frustration. Protective factors operate as well. For example, stable family functioning can prevent early temperamental difficulties from developing later into behavioral disorders.

SCHOOL-AGE (6–12 YEARS)

The *Latency Stage* in the elementary school years was called this by Freud because of the relative lack of sexual drives, thought to be channeled into socially appropriate activities, such as school work, sports, and games. Erikson described this as the *Industry vs. Inferiority* stage, in which the child is busy creating, building, and accomplishing. There is the danger of a sense of inferiority and inadequacy if a child feels unable to compete with regard to life skills, such as sports, academics, and social skills. For this reason, it is essential to diagnose learning disorders and help children gain the help they need to deal with them. Children who suffer from undetected developmental difficulties in any area may suffer from lowered self-esteem, as they compare their lack of accomplishment to the accomplishments of their peers. This is the age of best friends.

The *Concrete Operations* stage of cognitive development is postulated by Piaget for the ages of 6 to 11. The child in this stage gains the cognitive skills needed for basic logic, an understanding of cause and effect, and can begin to appreciate the perspectives of others—precisely the abilities that are necessary to benefit from the grade-school curriculum. The acquisition of the concept of conservation of volume and quantity occurs in this stage. This is when a child can appreciate that a tall, thin beaker holds the same amount of water as a short, fat one when it is poured back and forth between the two.

The developmental challenges of school may be particularly difficult for the fearful child, the overactive or inattentive child, or the poorly socialized child. Children who lack social skill, who have cognitive, learning, or coordination difficulties, or lack the ability to sit and pay attention and to control impulses and emotions may be quite frustrated in school, and may suffer from negative feedback from teachers and peers. Children who are anxious may develop separation anxiety and school-related anxiety, usually demonstrated by "tummy aches" or other complaints of illness in the morning prior to school. Additionally, teasing or bullying by peers may traumatize a child. Sociofamilial risk factors include poverty, single-parent family, abuse, chaotic home environment, or lack of supervision. During the school years, the prevalence of psychiatric disorders of all types increases.

CLINICAL VIGNETTE

Sally is a 7-year-old girl who is refusing to go to school. Her teacher describes Sally as a rather anxious, but also very oppositional girl. She refuses to do her work, won't participate in group reading or discussion, and goes to the nurse frequently with vague aches and pains, stating that she is sick and must go home. Sally has started to say unkind things to her best friend as well. Upon close assessment, you find out that Sally is unable to read. You request testing—results suggest that she is quite bright, with a severe reading disability (which is particularly difficult, because her best friend is an avid reader). Once this is identified and addressed, the oppositional and avoidant behaviors begin to resolve.

ADOLESCENCE

Adolescence is the developmental phase that spans the transition from relatively complete, childlike reliance on parents to nearly complete self-reliance for managing one's own life. Adolescence starts with puberty, the physical changes that initiate sexual maturation. In girls, puberty typically begins between the ages of 8 and 13, and in boys between 10 and 14. Sexual maturity for both boys and girls has been classified by Tanner, from Stage 1 (preadolescent) to Stage 5 (fully sexually mature).

Freud termed adolescence the *Genital Phase,* in which there is a recapitulation of earlier phases. Identity formation, separation from the family, and the biological capacity for orgasm and the psychological capacity for true intimacy develop. Erikson's *Identity vs. Role Confusion* captures the developmental task of this stage. Identification with a peer group begins to supplant that of the family. While adolescents may be preoccupied with appearance and demonstrate moodiness and emotional reactivity, it is also a time when they are gaining a sense of more permanent personal identity, values, and goals.

For Piaget, cognitive growth in adolescence ushers in the *Formal Operations* stage. The adolescent gains metacognitive capacity—the ability to think about thinking. The ability to use hypothetical and deductive abstract reasoning and the elaboration of information processing emerge. Many adolescents begin to think more deeply about religion, philosophy, and purpose.

Although adolescence can be a very turbulent time for many, high levels of distress are not the norm. Epidemiological studies do support the premise that anxiety and depression rise steeply during adolescence, particularly among girls. The four most common causes of death in the United States for teenagers are accidents, suicide, homicide, and cancer. Risk-taking behavior, which is relatively common in adolescence, as well as experimentation with drinking and illicit drugs, increases the likelihood of serious accidents. Suicide rates are higher for White males than for non-White males or females, although suicide gestures and attempts are higher in females. Homicides and gun-related deaths are particularly high for adolescents of color.

Adolescence is a time of increased risk for the onset of serious psychiatric disorders. Incidence rates for a number of psychiatric illnesses either peak or display a significant increase during adolescence. These include depression, bipolar disorder, panic disorder, obsessive-compulsive disorder, anorexia and bulimia nervosa, substance abuse, antisocial behavior, and schizophrenia. Illness in adolescence may evolve from the combination of biological vulnerability and adversity in family and community environments. Adolescent affiliation with a "bad crowd" may be an influential, separate variable that is associated with delinquency and social adjustment problems later.

Protective factors (resilience) are "multi-determined" by the personality disposition of the teen, a supportive family, and an external support system. Good physical health, normal or high IQ, and economic advantage may also play a protective role.

The Psychiatric Evaluation

Essential Concepts
- Providing a comprehensive initial psychiatric evaluation is the cornerstone for all effective treatment planning.
- The psychiatric evaluation is typically initiated by adults, and engaging the child, as well, is essential.
- A comprehensive evaluation includes gathering information from multiple sources (parents/guardians, school, primary care provider, child, and others).
- Inventory strengths as well as deficits/areas of need.
- The assessment of parent and family functioning is integral to the evaluation.

The work of psychological healing begins in a safe place . . . The psychological safe place permits the individual to make spontaneous, forceful gestures and, at the same time, represents a community that both allows the gestures and is valued for its own sake."

—Lester Havens, M.D.
A Safe Place

The psychiatric evaluation of a child or adolescent is not just a diagnostic interview and checklist of DSM-IV symptoms. It is much more—forming a rapport with the patient and family, learning about the child's functioning in multiple domains and from multiple sources, and assessing the child's family functioning (or environmental match if the child or adolescent is not living in the home). I like to think of myself as "Sherlock Holmes" during this time. I use the more obvious clues (usually the presenting complaint) to begin the investigation, as well as "digging deeper" to understand the nature of the symptoms and behavior, and the biological, psychological, and social factors which are precipitating and maintaining the impairing symptoms.

BASIC PRINCIPLES

Special Considerations in Evaluating Children

The psychiatric evaluation of a child or adolescent has a number of important differences from that of an adult:

- The referral is typically requested by someone other than the patient. The child (or adolescent) may feel ashamed, angry, or convinced that the evaluation is a punishment for being "bad." Try to set the stage to be as nonjudgmental and collaborative as possible, giving the child as much control as is appropriate and safe.
- Children are not just little adults. Remember the developmental stages (Chapter 1) and what to expect of a child of each age.
- Different methods of collecting data and interviewing the child apply at different ages. The goal is to understand the child's inner world and perspective. Techniques may range from observing an infant–parent dyad, or using play to understand the preschool and young elementary school child, to talking directly about symptoms with the adolescent. Remember to alter the approach to fit the developmental needs of the child. Drawing may be a helpful adjunctive tool at any age.
- The assessment of parental and family functioning is crucial. It is not possible to conduct an adequate assessment without an understanding of important environmental characteristics and family relationships, as well as the child's response to them.
- Use multiple informants. It is important to know if the child is having difficulties in all contexts, or only specific ones (for example, doing well at home, but having behavioral difficulties at school). This may help clarify the nature of the difficulty and point to specific areas for remediation.
- Diagnoses are more complicated in children. Although children may technically be diagnosed with almost any DSM-IV diagnosis, the varying presentation of symptoms at different ages, the evolution of disorders, and the lack of diagnostic and etiological specificity for many symptoms (impulsivity and aggression, for example) make diagnoses more fluid and unclear. It should be clarified that the diagnosis may change over time. However, this should not delay intervention and treatment of disabling symptoms.

Defining the Purpose of the Evaluation

Although many components to a psychiatric evaluation are similar to that of adults, how it is conducted, what information you need to glean, and how the information is used may be very different. Before you start, consider the purpose of the evaluation and use this information to structure the evaluation to fit the reason. Possible referral sources include:

- Parents (recommended by school, friends, relatives, themselves)
- Legal guardian (or state custody)
- Schools—they are paying for an evaluation of a student about whom they have concerns
- Courts—the child has legal issues, custody issues

The dynamics of the evaluation and how and where you conduct it depend on *why* you are doing the evaluation.

 TIP

Most families and children are intimidated by the prospect of seeing a psychiatrist. Depending upon the reason for and source of referral, you may have more or less buy-in for the evaluation. Clarify the reason up front and be attuned to the reactions of the entire family to your meeting. If another agency has recommended the evaluation, the parents may be suspicious about the process. Never ignore these subtle (or not so subtle) cues.

CLINICAL VIGNETTE

I was conducting an evaluation for a school system of a child with learning issues and acting-out behavior. The first meeting with the parents sought to clarify the dynamics of the evaluation.

Interviewer:	Hello [shaking hand of each parent and sitting down]. You know that I am a child and adolescent psychiatrist and that I have been asked by the school system to evaluate your son?
Father:	Right [looking disgruntled].
Interviewer:	I notice that you look unhappy to be here. Perhaps we can review what I have been asked to do to be sure that this is what you want.

In this case, the parents had requested a therapeutic school for their son (a school placement which would be expensive for the district and would place him with other special-needs children). The school district disagreed and maintained he would be better served in his home school. The parents felt the psychiatrist was a "hired gun" to prove the school's view that the child could be programmed for within-the-home school. The parents felt coerced and helpless. Bringing that out early in the interview helped to identify a needed aspect of the consultation—addressing the school–parent tensions.

🌐 KEY POINT

Who is paying for the evaluation is not a minor detail. Being an expert witness for one or the other side of a court case can strongly influence the "spin" of the same information. Be clear with yourself and your referral source who your client is. If the school or other agency is asking for a hired gun, be clear with everyone what you do. I find that the "best interest of the child" model works best. I try to keep my assessments focused on what I believe will ultimately lead to a more healthy developmental outcome for the child.

Setting the Stage

Setting the stage before you even meet the child or family is critical. Different clinics or private practitioners do this in different ways. Parents are often intimidated by the prospect of the evaluation, and few have a good notion of what it will entail. Most clinics use written statements of policies and procedures. As a trainee, you should know what information is given to families about policies and familiarize yourself with these. The following information should be included in communication (either on the phone or in the first session) with the parents or guardians before you begin:

1. Who you are—parents and guardians frequently need clarification about what different mental health professionals do. Explain your training and area of expertise.
2. What the psychiatric evaluation entails—with whom you will meet, in what order, what you do in the sessions, and what other information is needed.

3. How long it will take—how many sessions, how long per session.
4. What it will cost—for the evaluation as well as for ongoing treatment afterwards, if required.
5. What they can expect at the end—recommendations: a written report, ongoing treatment, etc.
6. What your policies are (define for patients and their families)—how and when to contact you, what to do in the event of an emergency, who you have permission to contact about the patient (HIPAA-friendly release of information forms required), and how you deal with missed appointments. Review for whom the evaluation is being done (parents or other agency) and the extent of confidentiality.
7. What to tell the child or adolescent to prepare him or her for the appointment.

If you are in a clinic, much of this work will be done by the intake person. Reiterating the information above is needed to clarify the goals and expectations for the evaluation.

The most uncomfortable part of an entire encounter for the clinician tends to be talking about billing. Although working in a clinic may spare you this difficult task, it is still important to mention it—to reiterate what the billing procedure is. I remember only too vividly my first encounter with a new patient's family after graduation from training. The words "bill" and "payment" seemed to stick in my mouth. Once I finally made this part of my written and verbal policies, I got much better at it—and my patients were less anxious as well.

⚜ TIP

I recommend that for an evaluation of a child, you meet first with the parents or guardians. For an adolescent it may be advisable to meet with the parents and adolescent patient in the initial interview to allay concerns of collusion with the parents. It is important to meet with both parents (if they are married or not) whenever possible. This is helpful in terms of getting various perspectives, as well as understanding the nature of the parental interactions, and how they each relate to and understand their child. In the case of divorced parents, you may need to meet with each parent or step-parent group separately. Getting a sense of how the parents work (or don't work) together in raising the child is important.

TIP

Explain to parents what type of professional you are. Many parents may confuse a psychiatric evaluation with psychological testing. The following introduction to the parents may be helpful:

I am a child and adolescent psychiatrist (or fellow)—a medical doctor who specializes in understanding and treating emotional and behavioral problems of children and teenagers. Perhaps we can spend just a few minutes reviewing what I do and what you expect, to make sure we're on the same page.

[Ask at this point what the parents are hoping to achieve from the evaluation. Then give a brief description of the nature of the evaluation.]

I try to get the best understanding I can of your child and his/her strengths as well as areas in which he/she is having real difficulties. To understand and help your child, I need to talk to the people who know him/her best. That is you, as his/her family, of course. But I also find that information from the school, pediatrician, (any others) is helpful. I will also meet and get to know your child. I will talk to him/her about things that he/she likes and is good at, as well as to try to understand the reasons that he/she is having difficulties. For younger children, I also use play with toys or games as a way of getting to know and understand him/her.

It is helpful to mention that you use play as an evaluative (and later, perhaps, therapeutic) tool for younger children. Some parents will be confused and distressed when their child, who has been causing such chaos in the home, comes out of the office and reports, "It was fun! We just played."

Follow up with how many times you will meet and get Release of Information forms signed (be sure to follow Health Insurance Portability and Accountability Act [HIPAA] guidelines).

I will meet with you for (an hour) today. Then I will meet with your child for (50 minutes, how many times and when). With your permission (explain HIPPA and get releases signed) I will also get information from your pediatrician, school, (any prior treaters, protective services, if there is involvement, any others. Ask if there are other sources with whom you should speak).

And now, for the difficult part—billing, cancellation policy, confidentiality, feedback, and procedure for contacting you. As a trainee, the financial aspects of billing and cancellation may seem irrelevant, but there are important clinical benefits to being clear about expectations (fewer cancellations and no-shows and more treatment compliance) and important training benefits to practicing this skill.

As you know, *[review the clinic billing and cancellation procedure]. When my evaluation is complete, I will meet with you [review the recommendation feedback procedure. If there will be a report generated, or not, clarify that. Also clarify with whom you will share the information. If the entire evaluation is court-ordered or requested by another agency with which a report will be shared, be clear about that. Clarify the extent of confidentiality, or lack thereof, with the parents, as well as the child or adolescent. If the report is being done for the Court, there is no confidentiality. Even in a regular practice, confidentiality is limited if you feel the child or others are in danger—state that up front. Clarify the clinic procedure for contacting you—both regular communication and after hours or for emergencies.]*

Before you end the session, review with the parents what they will tell their child about the evaluation. Help them practice explaining this to their child in a manner that is supportive and nonblaming. I have had parents tell their child that they were going out for ice cream, only to end up in my office. Although I learned a great deal about how the parents deal with their willful child (grist for the mill), needless to say, it did not set an inviting stage for the child to engage with me.

 TIP

Define the boundaries of the clinical practice by stating up front how, when, and for what the patients (or their families) can and should contact you.

- Don't give out your home number.
- Use voicemail for all nonemergency matters, and state how often you check it.
- For more urgent matters, specify how to contact you (if you use the pager system, be clear about when they may use this). An answering service contacting you is often preferable, when possible. Specify if you are available after hours or if there is a physician on call who takes care of all emergency matters.
- When you are going on vacation, sign out your patients to a trusted colleague. Having a backup person who knows the basics of your cases will assist in effective coverage.

KEY POINT

Set the stage for negotiation. For example, with teenagers it is sometimes helpful to meet with him or her first, before the parents, or meet with him or her with the parents, in order to give the adolescent some control. Be explicit that each child and family is unique. Be clear about which areas are flexible (with whom and in what order you meet, for example), and which are not (procedures for safety, for example).

 TIP

When you first meet with the child or adolescent, have the parents join the initial minutes of the meeting to review the reason for the evaluation and what to expect. I usually ask patients for their understanding of why they are here to see me first, and try to come to some shared agreement.

CLINICAL VIGNETTE

Children and adolescents may be unclear and anxious about the nature of the evaluation and if they are in trouble or being manipulated. In this example, the concerns and conflicts of the 12-year-old girl and her parents are addressed directly:

Interviewer:	*What is your understanding about why you are here to see me today?*
Child:	*I don't know. Didn't my parents already tell you?*
Parent to child:	*Yes, you do! Don't you remember that we talked about it?*
Interviewer to child:	*You're right, I have met with your parents and we have talked. But it helps me to hear what your understanding is.*
Child:	*To make me be a sweet little girl [sarcastically].*
Interviewer:	*I see. So your parents made you come, and you really don't want to be here.*
Child:	*Duh!*

Interviewer to parent:	*Did you tell her that we are here to make her a sweet little girl?*
Parent:	*Of course not! We told her we want to help our family communicate more effectively.*
Child:	*Yeah—meaning that you should talk and I should listen.*
Interviewer:	*So, you both agree that communicating and getting along could use some work?*
Child:	*And it's not just me!*
Interviewer:	*I see. So maybe the whole family needs to work at learning to talk out disagreements?*
Child:	*Yeah!*

With the child's feeling of being coerced brought out into the open, she was more forthcoming and less defensive throughout the rest of the interview.

COMPONENTS OF THE PSYCHIATRIC EVALUATION

The child and adolescent psychiatric evaluation consists of at least three elements: 1) interview, information gathering, and basic assessment of the family or primary caretakers/legal guardians; 2) interview/assessment of the child or adolescent; 3) information from other sources (primary care physician, school, or others, as needed). The logistics of how these three elements are obtained may vary. In my ideal initial evaluation of a new patient whom I may take on in treatment, I first meet with the parents or guardians (together, if possible, even if they are divorced), then with the entire family unit (family that lives in the home with the identified patient), then with the child or adolescent one or two times. I will call the other informants (school, primary care physician, etc.) and then plan a feedback meeting with the parents to discuss findings and recommendations. In real life, it may be impractical to obtain an evaluation in this manner. However, I find that meeting the entire family can be very instructive in terms of understanding dynamics and formulating appropriate and effective therapeutic interventions. It also sets the stage for the difficulties not being the "fault" of the identified patient in isolation (Table 2.1 lists components of a through psychiatric evaluation and Table 2.2

TABLE 2.1. Components of a Thorough Psychiatric Evaluation

- Referral source—clarify who is requesting the assessment and for what purpose
- Chief complaint(s) and goals of the assessment
- Context—find out in what context(s) problems occur
- Multiple informants—incorporate information from the primary care physician, school or child care, both parents or guardians, mental health providers, and any other involved agencies, e.g., juvenile justice, child welfare. Get Release of Information forms signed to speak to each.
- Patient interview/Mental status examination—interview the child or adolescent alone. Use open-ended questions and try to ascertain the child or adolescent's perspective of the issues. With young children, observing and describing play is more helpful. The Mental Status Exam may be more observational and interactive than with adults.
- Family Evaluation—see the entire family together whenever possible. If not the whole family, seeing the child or adolescent and parents together is helpful to clarify family dynamics.
- Medical Evaluation—obtain the medical history and talk to the primary care physician. Clarify if any further medical workup is required, e.g., EEG to rule out seizures, neuroimaging, screening labs to rule out potential medical causes, ECG or other appropriate labs prior to a medication trial. Table 2.2 summarizes medical factors that may have a psychiatric presentation to be considered.
- Psychoeducational testing, if needed, to rule out learning disability and intellectual impairment (at times, neuropsychological testing to assess executive functioning and more subtle or complex deficits), projective testing, speech and language assessments, or other evaluations may be indicated to clarify the nature of the presenting symptoms.
- Rating scales (such as Conners for ADHD, Beck Depression Inventory for depression, etc.) to assess the number and severity of symptoms. Baseline and follow-up rating scales are helpful in monitoring.
- School functioning—talking to teachers and school personnel may be very helpful in understanding the difficulties (as well as strengths) of the child. Be sure to ask about peer and teacher interactions, how he or she deals with transitions or changes, learning style and motivation, as well as overall academic level. A classroom observation may be helpful.

TABLE 2.2. Medical Factors That May Have a Psychiatric Presentation

Medications/toxic/ drug-induced	Corticosteroids, benzodiazepines, amphetamines, anticholinergics, hallucinogens, antihypertensives, asthma medications, narcotics, lead exposure
Genetic	Fragile X syndrome, Wilson disease, Prader-Willi syndrome, Klinefelter syndrome
Infectious/Immunologic	Lyme disease, infectious mononucleosis, HIV/AIDS, tuberculosis, neoplasm, lupus erythematosis and other autoimmune disorders, chronic fatigue syndrome, PANDAS (pediatric autoimmune neuropsychiatric disorders associated with streptococcal infection)
Neurologic	Epilepsy, migraines, central nervous system tumor, traumatic brain injury, anoxia, demyelinating processes
Endocrinologic	Hypo- and hyperthyroidism, diabetes, hypopituitarism, androgenization, Cushing disease, adrenal insufficiency
Other	Hypoglycemia, electrolyte abnormalities, uremia

details medical factors that should be considered in a workup of the etiology of psychiatric symptoms).

Appendix 1a gives an outline of the components of a child and adolescent psychiatric evaluation report.

Family Assessment

Accurate psychiatric assessment and effective treatment of an individual child must involve an examination of family process. Family process refers to the repetitive patterns of interaction between members. The definition of "family" may be broad, but understanding the bonds and processes within a family context will help you more fully understand the child. No child lives in isolation, and the context and dynamics of the child's nurturing environment may serve a role as a primary protective or primary risk factor (or both). Failure to recognize the importance of family process may prevent the initiation of appropriate treatment interventions and may place a psychiatric clinician in the role of unwitting participant in an unhealthy family system.

Family theorists vary on the type of approach used to assess family functioning. I find the following most useful.

Family genogram. In the initial meeting with the parents I ask about a basic family history. This may be most efficiently done in a genogram. The genogram, as presented by McGoldrick, is a practical and useful framework for understanding family patterns and mapping out how family members are biologically and legally related to one another over a series of several generations. I include any psychiatric, learning, medical or substance use issues, history of abuse or neglect, and legal issues next to each circle (female) or square (male) person in the genogram. Usually grandparents and subsequent generations are sufficient. Ask about cultural and religious background, as well.

Family diagnostic interview. Different clinicians do this in different ways. I use the following format:

> *Greeting*: This is the time to set the stage that you are interested in the entire family and how they get along, not just the "identified patient" (who may not turn out to be the primary difficulty). Example: "Hello. It is so nice to get to meet your whole family." [*Have each sibling say his or her name and age*]. You may ask what their understanding of the meeting is. A statement such as the following may be helpful: "I understand that we are meeting here today to help me get to know your family and how you get along together."
>
> *Typical day*: Ask the family to describe a typical weekday. Who gets up first? How do they organize to get ready for school, work, etc.? Who goes where? How do they like school, job, etc.? When do they get home? Do they eat dinner together? What is a usual evening like? Where does each person sleep?
>
> *What they like to do together*: Ask the family in general to say what they like to do together. I try to be sure that each member (if old enough) contributes.
>
> *What they like best about their family*: Again, be sure to hear from all members.
>
> *What they would like to change or be different in their family*: Let each family member answer.

TIP

If there are young ones (preschool or kindergarten age), set up some simple toys in the circle (crayons and paper can be quite sufficient) and allow them to play as you talk; they usually are listening intently and know what is going on. Be sure to include the little ones, if they can talk. It may be the youngest member who has the most insight (the 4-year-old is often the one that "spills the beans" about dysfunctional family secrets) and gives a good overall sense of the family's strengths, vulnerabilities, and areas of need.

Family Functioning Rating Scales

A variety of rating scales are available to help clinicians assess family functioning. These may already be used in your clinic. If not, examples of family rating scales include:

Family Environment Scale (FES) by Moos and Moos—measures family cohesion, expressiveness, conflict, independence, and achievement

Family Assessment Devise (FAD) by Miller—based on a problem-centered model and examines the structure of families regarding problem-solving abilities, communication, roles, and general functioning

Family Adaptability Cohesion Evaluation Scale (FACES III) by Olson et al. —a self-report instrument that describes family processes such as negotiations, family roles, boundaries, coalitions, decision making, assertiveness, and discipline

Family Formulation

This need not be formal but will integrate into your overall formulation of the child's biopsychosocial functioning at the completion of the assessment. Consider overall family functioning, problem-solving abilities, intrafamily communications and boundaries, behavioral control, affective processes, and family cohesion and adaptability as areas that impact each family member.

Patient Interview: The Mental Status Examination

For children and adolescents, the mental status examination components may be gathered through direct questioning, play activities, or observations during the session.

- Appearance and behavior: grooming, size, type of dress, dysmorphic features, bruises, scars or injuries, eye contact
- Ability to cooperate and engage with assessment
- Social relatedness
- Speech and language: fluency, volume, rate, and language skills (appropriateness for developmental level, articulation issues, social speech)
- Motor function: activity level, coordination, attention, frustration tolerance, impulsivity, tics and mannerisms
- Mood and affect: neurovegetative symptoms, manic symptoms, range and appropriateness of affects
- Thought process and content: psychotic symptoms (hallucinations, delusions, thought disorder)
- Anxiety: fears and phobias, obsessions or compulsions, post-traumatic anxiety, separation difficulties
- Conduct symptoms: oppositionality, conduct symptoms, aggression (verbal or physical)
- Trauma history: physical or sexual abuse, neglect
- Assessment of risk: suicidal thoughts or behavior, self-abusive behavior, thoughts or plans to harm others, risk-taking behaviors, sexual behaviors, internet usage, legal issues, cigarette, substance or alcohol experimentation/use
- Cognitive functioning: overall assessment of developmentally appropriate vocabulary, fund of knowledge, drawings
- Insight and judgment: acknowledgment of having a problem, judgment for hypothetical situations

Rating Scales/Assessment Instruments

Rating scales range from systematized questionnaires that assess psychiatric symptoms in general to those that probe specific areas of difficulty in depth. Advantages of using rating scales include their assisting the clinician in the systematic evaluation of the child, including detecting problems that are clinically significant but not part of the presenting problem. Some adolescents may reveal concerns in writing that they do not verbalize. Disadvantages of using rating scales include the time needed to complete them, the feeling of being "check-listed," and clinicians' tendency to over-rely on rating scales for diagnosis. Rating scales are adjunctive tools used to complement a diagnostic evaluation, not replace it.

With children and adolescents, the rating scales may be completed by the patient or by parents or teachers. Additionally, semistructured diagnostic interviews (Diagnostic Interview for Children, or DISC; children's version of Schizophrenia and Affective Disorders Scale, or K-SADS) are typically used for research purposes, but may be used clinically for diagnostic clarification.

Appendix 2 gives a summary of some commonly used rating scales.

Clinical Formulation and Diagnosis

I consider the clinical formulation and diagnosis the critical skill that characterizes child and adolescent psychiatry. It is the integration of the complex and sometimes disparate information gleaned from the evaluation above, putting it in a context to understand the child's behavior and to clarify the treatment focus and appropriate interventions. There are two primary formulation prototypes: biopsychosocial and the 4 Ps.

Biopsychosocial formulation. This is still the most commonly used formulation type for the Board examinations. It interweaves biological vulnerabilities (prenatal, birth, early temperament, development, genetic predispositions/family history, medical and neurological disorders), psychological factors (personality, psychological issues and attributions, defense mechanisms, developmental stage tasks), and social/environmental contributors (family/interpersonal, socioenvironmental, trauma, and cultural factors) to postulate an understanding of what brings the child or adolescent to this point in life. With this understanding, the most focused and effective treatment recommendations can be formulated.

The 4 Ps. Another useful method of formulation is the 4 Ps, as proposed by Barker.

1. Predisposing—those factors that render the child vulnerable to a disorder
2. Precipitating—stressors or developmental factors that are associated with the emergence or worsening of symptoms
3. Perpetuating—factors that maintain the disabling symptoms
4. Protective—strengths and assets that may be accessed to promote more healthy adjustment and diminish the severity of symptoms

Each of the 4 Ps may be described along the following dimensions: (a) biological/constitutional (including prenatal, birth, early temperament, and genetic vulnerabilities), (b) psychological/personality/temperament, (c) family/interpersonal, and (d) socioenvironmental.

The formulation need not be lengthy, but it is important. The formulation serves to integrate and synthesize the information obtained into a coherent understanding of the multiple factors which are likely contributing to or diminishing symptom severity. It is this understanding that informs the diagnosis, prognosis, and treatment recommendations.

Diagnosis. Diagnosis is typically given in Axis I-V as recommended in the DSM-IV.

Axis I	*Clinical disorders*
	Other conditions that may be a focus of clinical attention
Axis II	*Personality disorders*
	Mental retardation
Axis III	*General medical conditions*
Axis IV	*Psychosocial and environmental problems*
Axis V	*Global assessment of functioning*

COMMUNICATING FINDINGS AND RECOMMENDATIONS

Feedback to the Family

The evaluation is not complete until findings are communicated to parents, the child, and/or other referring agencies. The purpose of the feedback is to help provide an empathic understanding of the etiology of the difficulties and strengths of the youngster assessed, and to communicate this diagnostic understanding in a manner that will help provide a clear focus for therapeutic interventions. Avoid psychiatric jargon when possible.

Be sure to set aside sufficient time to explain the rationale for the diagnoses given and treatment recommendations. If you give the diagnoses in all five axes, they will need to be explained. For purposes of the family, axis I and II are usually sufficient. If you have provisional diagnoses, be clear that you are not sure. I often tell parents that children frequently don't fit neatly into our diagnostic categories, and each child is unique. The formulation may be more helpful than definitive diagnoses in understanding and helping the child.

Feedback to Other Agencies

Feedback given to schools or other agencies will be focused primarily on the referral questions, although a comprehensive evaluation is typically conducted to answer those questions. If dangerousness is a concern, this should be explored in detail, including precipitating factors, chronic stressors, and previous history of violence. Recommendations should emphasize the most practical, helpful, and necessary treatment approach that is in the best interest of the child. Crucial information should be elucidated, while maintaining sensitivity to family and personal information which is not relevant to the evaluation. Recommendations should be clear and as specific and concrete as possible.

 TIP

Keep feedback in lay language that is nonjudgmental, sensitive, and practical. Parents may be very anxious about hearing what is wrong with their child (and family). Remember that very little of the information you say will be retained, especially if there is an emotional component. Usually feedback is given to the parents first, but, depending on the nature of the problem and the developmental level of the child, it may be appropriate for the child or adolescent to be there. If the child is there, talk to him or her directly about the findings. Be sure to provide a written report or succinct summary for the parents and/or ongoing dialogue, discussion, and psychoeducation regarding your findings and recommendations.

RECOMMENDATIONS FOR TREATMENT

Recommendations should flow naturally from your formulation and diagnoses. Just as the formulation is biopsychosocial, so are treatment recommendations. Begin with any further assessments required (neurological, medical, and/or psychoeducational assessments) for more specificity of treatment and diagnosis.

Selection of appropriate treatment is based on multiple factors, including diagnosis and symptom severity, acute and ongoing risk of harm, capacity of the family to support treatment and provide a safe environment, capacity of the child to engage in and use interactive treatment approaches, and availability of treatment options in the community.

A comprehensive treatment plan should include consideration of the intensity of treatment required for the child in a systems-based manner:

1. Child is at imminent risk and requires acute hospitalization
2. Child needs higher level of care than can be provided safely in the home, but is not at imminent risk—residential treatment, group home, subacute temporary residential stabilization, therapeutic foster home, safe home, etc.

3. Child can be maintained safely in the home only with intensive wraparound services—in-home behavioral services, partial hospitalization or after-school therapeutic program, intensive case management, etc.
4. Child requires regular outpatient therapeutic services
   a. Individual therapy (cognitive behavioral therapy (CBT), insight-oriented, supportive, interpersonal therapy (ITP), dialectic behavioral therapy (DBT), anger management, etc.)
   b. Psychotropic medication for treatment of psychiatric symptoms that are amenable to medication
   c. Group therapy (therapy group, social and coping skills groups, DBT group)
   d. Family therapy (regular family therapy, parent management training, parent psychoeducation, multisystemic treatment (MST), couples therapy, divorce mediation and conflict resolution, or parents accessing needed treatment for themselves)
5. Other adjunctive services
   a. School services (special education or Section 504) for emotional, attentional, and/or learning issues, including in-school counseling, therapeutic interventions and services within mainstream classroom, special education classroom, or out-of-district placement at a school specializing in working with children with emotional, social, and/or behavioral difficulties
   b. Speech therapy for language problems (including social conversation) as appropriate to the child's difficulties
   c. State Protective Service involvement as needed for suspected abuse or neglect or for voluntary services for the family
   d. Legal involvement accessed by the family to help monitor a child with severe out-of-control behavior
   e. Other supports, such as Big Brother or Sister, mentoring programs, respite home, recreational therapy, and pet therapy.

 TIP

Many parents ask if their child will "grow out of" the difficulties or express concerns that if they start medications their child will require medications for his or her lifetime. I take the tact that we cannot predict the future, but we do know that developmental scars may remain when a child does not receive the help he or she requires academically, socially, emotionally, or behaviorally. Not all children will require intensive or long-term treatment for these issues, but it is crucial that they be addressed and taken seriously to allow the child to develop as optimally as possible.

CLINICAL VIGNETTE

Parents brought their 10-year-old fourth-grade son for evaluation because of increasing behavioral problems at home and at school. He had always had difficulties in school—fidgeting, calling out in class, being disorganized and disruptive. He had begun to act out behaviorally in school when called on in class. He spoke to his teacher in a disrespectful manner and did not complete his work. At home he refused to do his homework and became angry and shouted, slammed doors, and stomped off when his parents tried to insist. On evaluation, he seemed easily distracted and very defensive and difficult to engage about any perceived inadequacies. A Conner's Scale of attention deficit hyperactivity disorder symptoms completed by the teacher and parents suggested a high level of symptoms. Further investigation revealed a family history of ADHD and learning disabilities. A recommendation was made for psychoeducational testing, which demonstrated above-average overall cognitive ability with a specific reading disability. In formulation, the *predisposing* factors (family genetics for ADHD and a reading disability) and *precipitating* factors (increasing expectations in school and at home as he got older) were manifested in oppositional and defiant behavior to ward off feelings of inadequacy academically and in his inability to control his impulses. This was *perpetuated* by a family and school stance of punitive consequences for misbehavior and unreasonably high expectations for this otherwise bright boy. *Protective* factors included above-average overall cognitive skills, concerned parents, athletic abilities, and some friends. Recommendations were for a reading tutor and special assistance with reading, including the use of tapes, oral tests, extra time for tests, and modifications of assignments. Special accommodations for the ADHD symptoms, including preferential seating near the teacher, subtle cues to gain and focus attention, and organizational assistance were recommended, along with the recommendation for a stimulant medication trial. Parent counseling and psychoeducation and child anger management training were also suggested. When these interventions were implemented, the child made significant improvements.

II

AXIS I DISORDERS USUALLY FIRST DIAGNOSED IN INFANCY, CHILDHOOD, OR ADOLESCENCE

Developmental Disorders
· ·

Mental Retardation

Essential Concepts
- Assessment and clarification of learning, cognitive, and developmental disorders are essential to providing appropriate interventions
- Early diagnosis and appropriate and intensive interventions for developmental delay improve prognosis
- A systems-based approach is needed to work with developmentally disabled children and families
- Inventory strengths as well as deficits and areas of need
- Other psychiatric disorders (mood, anxiety, behavioral) are more common in children with mental retardation.

Many children with mental retardation are never referred to a child and adolescent psychiatrist or mental health professional of any kind. Pediatricians, family practitioners, pediatric neurologists, special educators, speech and language and physical or occupational therapists tend to provide services for these children. Birth to Three Early Intervention provides crucial services in the early identification and early treatment intervention of children with developmental and cognitive disorders. However, trainees and practitioners in child and adolescent psychiatry need to be comfortable and competent working with children with these disorders, as the comorbidity with other psychiatric disorders of mood, anxiety, and behavior are extremely high. Working with children with developmental disabilities requires a high degree of comfort and sophistication in collaborating in a multidisciplinary system of care to provide the full range of services needed to optimize outcome.

BASIC PRINCIPLES

It should not be assumed that children with special learning needs will have other psychiatric difficulties. However, children with mental retardation have a three to four times higher incidence of other psychiatric disorders than children with average cognitive skills. Mentally retarded children are at high risk for social ostracism. Additionally, the neuropathology underlying the learning or cognitive dysfunction may contribute to certain aberrant behaviors. Executive and problem-solving skills are impaired concomitantly with the overall cognitive delay.

 KEY POINT

Individuals with mental retardation consist of a widely variable group of children. Each child must be individually evaluated regarding special learning needs, as well as emotional level of functioning, to formulate an individualized educational (and possibly mental health) plan. Remember to assess strengths as well as deficits.

DIAGNOSTIC CRITERION AND EPIDEMIOLOGY

Mental retardation is diagnosed on Axis II in the DSM multiaxial diagnostic scheme. The diagnosis of mental retardation requires the concomitant impairment in cognitive functioning, as well as impairments in adaptive functioning (person's effectiveness in meeting age-expected standards in communication, self-care, home living, social/interpersonal skills, use of community resources, self-direction, functional academic skills, work, leisure, health and safety). It is estimated that about 1% of the population meet these criteria. Tables 3.1 and 3.2 define the severity levels of mental retardation, as well as the possible etiologies.

COMORBID MENTAL DISORDERS

It is estimated that 30 to 70% of mentally retarded children also suffer from a psychiatric disorder. Neurobiological as well as environmental factors (stigmatization, feeling of failure in school) put these children at very high risk. The most common associated mental disorders are attention deficit

TABLE 3.1. Mental Retardation (Axis II except Borderline on Axis I)

Severity	Approximate IQ Range
Borderline	71–84
Mild	50–55 to 70
Moderate	35–40 to 50–55
Severe	20–25 to 35–40
Profound	Below 20–25

hyperactivity disorder, pervasive developmental disorders, mood and anxiety disorders, stereotypic movement disorder, and mental disorders due to a general medical condition (such as dementia due to head trauma).

There are a few mental retardation symptoms that are associated with specific genetic syndromes and place a child at high risk of specific psychiatric disorders. Individuals with: Down syndrome are at higher risk for developing Alzheimer-type dementia; fragile X syndrome are at increased risk for ADHD and social phobia; Prader-Willi syndrome frequently demonstrate hyperphagia and obsessive and compulsive symptoms; William's syndrome have high risk for anxiety disorders and ADHD.

TABLE 3.2. Etiology of Mental Retardation

Type	Description
Hereditary	Familial or sporadic chromosomal aberrations
Early alterations (embryonic development)	Prenatal damage due to infection, toxins, and substance abuse, or etiology unknown
Pregnancy, perinatal problems	Fetal malnutrition, prematurity, hypoxia, viral and other infections, and trauma
Medical conditions of infancy	Infections (esp. CNS), traumas, poisoning (e.g., lead) Other illnesses (e.g., thyroid, cancers and treatment)
Environmental influences	Severe early neglect or abuse, malnutrition

TIP

Medications may be used to treat the comorbid psychiatric disorder in children and adolescents with cognitive delays who demonstrate psychiatric disorders which may benefit from the medication. However, in general "start lower and go slower" on initial dosages and medication titrations, as there may be increased sensitivity to side effects.

KEY POINT

The primary goal of treatment is to improve the quality of life of a child or adolescent with cognitive delay, and help him or her achieve the highest level of functioning possible.

KEY POINT

The role of the child and adolescent psychiatrist in working with individuals with mental retardation was specified by the American Academy of Child and Adolescent Psychiatry as 1) provision of clinical services; 2) prevention of mental disorders through early diagnosis and provision of emotional supports to the child and family; 3) research; 4) learning skills that are also useful in the practice of psychiatry in general.

CLINICAL VIGNETTE

Jason is an active, cute and engaging 5-year-old boy who is in kindergarten at his local elementary school. He was in a family day care prior to beginning kindergarten. He is an only child of parents who are hard-working and caring, but neither of whom received a high school education, having dropped out and then conceived Jason when the mother was 17 years of age. His mother had used substances (alcohol and marijuana), but stated that she stopped when she found out she was pregnant.

Jason made a reasonable adjustment to kindergarten socially, although the teacher has reported that he is inattentive, easily distractible, and refuses to do his letter, number, and other work. When she insists, he tends to become oppositional and defiant (refusing or pushing and hitting her) or to scribble and not put forth good effort. He is referred to you for evaluation of possible ADHD. On examination, Jason seems delayed in his fine motor skills and speech, with some immature articulation as well as sparse speech. The pediatrician noted early developmental delays in all spheres. You request cognitive and academic evaluations, which demonstrate a full-scale IQ on the Wexler Preschool and Primary Scales of Intelligence (WPPSI) of 62 (the mean is 100), with preacademic skills similarly low. Additionally, his adaptive functioning is delayed in communication, self-care, home and community living, and functional academic skills. He is diagnosed with mild mental retardation. You recommend special education services to address his learning needs. When he is provided with periods of the day with small group or individual attention for his academic subjects, his behaviors improve. However, a high degree of inattention and distractibility still seems to be impairing his ability to learn. You begin a low dose (2.5 mg and titrate up to 5 mg in morning and at noon) of methylphenidate, which seems to be effective for his inattention. Jason's behavior and effort improve. A multidisciplinary treatment group, which includes speech and language and special education services, the pediatrician, in-home service providers to help his parents provide an enriched environment and structure at home, and you as the child and adolescent psychiatrist provide an array of services for this child and family, to the benefit of the child's functioning. Three years later, his follow-up cognitive testing suggests a full-scale IQ of 69, with educational functioning in the mid-70s. Adaptive functioning and overall behavioral control have also improved.

✦ KEY POINT

Although psychological tests are becoming normed to a wider range of cultures and ethnicities, clinicians need to be sensitive to these issues in interpreting tests. Test results may not be accurate in children whose primary language is not English. Additionally, preschool children's testing may not be as reliable (remain the same over time) as for older children.

Assessment

The individual administration of both a standardized cognitive test (such as the Wechsler Intelligence scale for children, WISC-IV; the Kaufman Assessment Battery for Children, K-ABC; the Stanford Binet Intelligence Scale 4th edition, or others) *and* a measure of adaptive functioning (such as the Vineland Adaptive Behavior Scale) is required for diagnosis of mental retardation. The tests should be administered in the child's dominant language whenever possible and estimates of the validity of test administration considered. If the child is nonverbal, there are tests (such as the Comprehensive Test of Nonverbal Intelligence, C-TONI or the Leiter International Performance Scale) that may be used.

Medical evaluation and collaboration with the primary care physician is an important aspect to the evaluation. Medical evaluation includes a careful prenatal and developmental history, family history, neurological evaluation, laboratory screening (thyroid, lead, and routine labs, as well as investigation of rarer inborn errors of metabolism, VDRL, and chromosomal analysis, as appropriate), as well as possibly brain imaging (MRI) and electroencephalogram (EEG) to rule out seizures.

The differential diagnosis of mental retardation includes hearing or visual impairment, autism and other pervasive developmental disorders, learning disabilities or borderline cognitive functioning, and severe early neglect or abuse.

Treatment

Early detection and developmentally sensitive multimodal treatment are required for optimal outcomes. Another key element is parent guidance and support, as the diagnosis of mental retardation is quite devastating to parents. Birth to Three services can assist with the early assessment and intervention. Recommended services typically include speech and language therapy, physical or occupational therapy, early stimulation, advocacy for services, educational and environmental planning, behavior management, and teaching of functional and self-care skills. Standard therapies are used for psychiatric comorbidities, with the careful and judicious use of medication, as appropriate. In-home behavioral services and respite care opportunities may also be indicated. It is important that the services are well coordinated and that there is good multidisciplinary collaboration in the care of children with complex and multiple disabilities.

Prognosis is variable, depending on the type and severity of the mental retardation. In general, children with mild mental retardation (85% of those with MR) can anticipate gaining academic skills at about the sixth-grade level, with the ability to hold a job and function with minimal supports in the community. Prognosis is markedly improved with early intervention and education, a focus on job skills and independent living skills, good medical care of physical and psychiatric illness, and a supportive environment.

▼ TIP

Many child and adolescent psychiatrists never gain the skills and comfort level to work with severely mentally retarded children. Odd or unpredictable behavior may be off-putting, deficits in language skills make diagnosis and treatment especially challenging, and the risk of aggressive behavior in some children may be frightening. However, I have found working with this group of children to be highly gratifying. Interventions can be quite helpful. Your child and adolescent psychiatry expertise in providing assistance to the family, the school, and the child may make a substantial positive influence on the child's prognosis.

Learning Disorders

Essential Concepts
- A learning disability is a significant discrepancy between assessed cognitive ability and assessed academic achievement.
- Learning disorders of reading, mathematics, and written language are defined in the Diagnostic and Statistical Manual (DSM-IV-TR).
- Children with learning disorders have a high prevalence of comorbid emotional and behavioral difficulties.
- Early identification and intervention are essential for optimal prevention of further learning, emotional, and behavioral problems.

Identification and intervention of learning disabilities (LDs) in children is primarily the function of the educational system. However, children with LD have many risk factors for emotional and behavioral difficulties: frustration at school, poor self-esteem, criticism by adults who don't understand the disability, and biological vulnerabilities. It is these secondary disorders that prompt consultation to a mental health professional.

Early detection and specialized tutoring and teaching techniques may be quite helpful in improving prognosis. Additionally, it is essential that the child, his or her parents, and school personnel have a good understanding of the nature of the disability, to minimize the risk of the child "feeling stupid," academic failure, and criticism for "not trying" or being "lazy," which may erode self-esteem and precipitate emotional and behavioral difficulties. Because children with learning disabilities are usually bright, they are more cognizant of their difficulties than individuals with more pervasive cognitive and learning issues. It is heartbreaking to hear a child call himself "stupid" when he is quite bright but unable to read.

BASIC PRINCIPLES

It should not be assumed that children with special learning needs will have other psychiatric difficulties. However, children with learning disorders have a high incidence of psychiatric difficulties. An estimated 15 to 25% of children with reading disability will meet criteria for ADHD. School avoidance, depressive moods (14–32%) and anxiety disorders are also common. Overall, girls with LDs are more likely to suffer from internalizing symptoms and boys from externalizing symptoms. Additionally, learning disorders frequently co-occur. It is common for a child to demonstrate more than one learning disorder or a concomitant language disorder.

Diagnostic Criterion and Epidemiology

All learning disorders are diagnosed by the administration of an individually administered standardized measure of intelligence (such as the Wechsler Intelligence Scale for Children—WISC) and an individually administered achievement test (such as the Wechsler Individual Achievement Test—WIAT). If the academic achievement in a given area (reading, mathematics, or written language) is substantially below that expected given the person's chronological age, education, and measured intelligence, and is functionally impairing, a learning disorder may be diagnosed. The Individuals with Disability Education Act (IDEA PL 94-142) provides for services under the classification of Specific Learning Disability. For a child to be eligible for special education services, a statistically significant difference of at least 1.5 to 2 standard deviations between assessed academic achievement and cognitive ability must exist.

Table 4.1 chronicles the characteristics of the LDs.

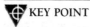 **KEY POINT**

Child and adolescent psychiatrists and other mental health professionals can provide essential psychoeducation to parents, school personnel, and the child about the nature of the learning difficulty and advocate for essential educational services. Reframing the task to that of effective teaching and learning (as opposed to a misbehavior or basic flaw) improves a child's self-esteem. Treating coexisting ADHD, if it is present, may also improve the child's ability to focus and learn. Using the child's strengths to find and promote areas in which he or she excels improves self-image and sense of worth.

TABLE 4.1. The Learning Disorders

	Reading Disorder (RD)	Mathematics Disorder (MD)	Written Language Disorder (WD)
Clinical features	Dyslexia Deficit in phonological awareness—processing sounds (phonemes) that make up language Difficulty with rapid and fluent word retrieval	Two problem areas: Basic math processes and procedural difficulties Problem with working memory and executive function skills Lower visual spatial skills	Requires higher-order cognitive and executive functions Requires handwriting, spelling, and ability to express ideas through text
Epidemiology	3–10% of population Male 4: Female 1	1–5% of school-age children No gender difference	Estimated 15–20% of school-age children
Etiology	Familial and genetic Reversed asymmetry of brain activation when reading Environmental effects	Familial and genetic Commonly co-occurs with another LD Inferior left prefrontal cortex implicated	Unclear and multi-determined

(Continued)

TABLE 4.1. The Learning Disorders (*continued*)

	Reading Disorder (RD)	Mathematics Disorder (MD)	Written Language Disorder (WD)
Differential diagnosis	Vision or hearing problems MR Cultural or language factors Environment	50% of children with MD also have RD	Frequently coexists with other LDs Rule out cultural, environmental, and cognitive issues
Clinical course	Matthew effects—accumulated disadvantage of not being able to read fluently 75% with some persistent symptoms 40% school dropout rate	Chronic and persistent through school Early intervention helpful Lack of data on clinical course	Early intervention improves prognosis Unknown course
Treatment	Intense, high-quality instruction on phonemic awareness and phonics	Techniques to increase computational and math problem-solving skills (validated)	Use of a consistent framework for writing Organizational skills

OTHER SKILLS DISORDERS

In addition to the learning disorders, there are a variety of developmental skills disorders described in DSM. Motor skills disorder (Developmental Coordination Disorder) and the communication disorders (Expressive Language Disorder, Mixed Receptive-Expressive Language Disorder, Phonological Disorder, Stuttering and Communication Disorder, NOS) are developmental disorders characterized by skills (motor or language) which are substantially below those expected given the child's age and measured intelligence. As with other developmental disorders, early identification and intensive evidence-based intervention improve prognosis.

CLINICAL VIGNETTE

Brianna is a bright 6-year-old girl who is in the first grade. She loved kindergarten, but has begun to complain of stomachaches before school and to state that she is too ill to go to school. The teacher states that Brianna has friends and seems to enjoy her peers. However, she is very resistant to doing her school work. She refuses to participate in her small reading group and will not read aloud, as the other children do. This oppositionality is becoming increasingly problematic. When the teacher attempted to test her skill level, Brianna refused to participate. Upon the recommendation of the pediatrician, Brianna received full cognitive and intellectual testing. Although her intellectual functioning was overall in the high average range, her reading ability was in the deficient range. The diagnosis of a reading disability was made. Sharing this information with the parents, teacher, and Brianna helped to reframe her symptoms. She was told that her brain was very smart, but that her brain had a harder time learning to read than many other children (although she was reassured that other children also have reading disorders). This meant that she had to work harder to learn to read than other children, and it was not her fault—it did not mean that she was "dumb" (as she called herself). Brianna began to receive 30 minutes daily of individualized training with the REACH system (a comprehensive phonetic skills teaching system). As she began to learn to read, her complaints about going to school and oppositionality began to subside. Brianna was artistic, and her artwork was displayed (with that of some other children) in the art exhibit area, much to her delight.

5 Pervasive Developmental Disorders: The Autism Spectrum Disorders

Essential Concepts
- The essential feature of the pervasive developmental disorders is abnormal social development and relatedness.
- Early detection and early intervention improve prognosis.
- Some children may be diagnosed before 1 year of age.
- Treatment should be multimodal and multidimensional.
- Anxiety and other psychiatric disorders may complicate prognosis and treatment.

Pervasive developmental disorders (PDDs) are also referred to as the autism spectrum disorders (ASDs). There are five disorders in this category: autism, Asperger disorder, Rett disorder, childhood disintegrative disorder, and pervasive developmental disorder, not otherwise specified (PDD, NOS). The core feature of the PDDs is an abnormal relatedness and social development. Although cognitive and motor development are often also affected, it is the manner of relating and communicating that is the sine qua non of the disorders.

These are tragic yet fascinating disorders. Although the movie *Rainman* was fiction, individuals with ASDs may be high functioning in many ways, but experience an extreme need for sameness and routine, lack of flexibility, inability to read social cues and interact in a reciprocal manner, and odd speech. The term "spectrum" is sometimes used to denote the fact that the level of impairment and disability can be quite variable.

At one time, individuals with ASDs were thought to be resistant to intervention. We now know that early multimodal and multidimensional treatment may markedly improve prognosis. Support for the family, in addition to the child, is also required. Psychiatrists work within a system of care to provide needed services for a child and his or her family.

BASIC PRINCIPLES

From the earliest description of autism by Leo Kanner in 1943, the disorder has been studied widely to ascertain the etiology and effective treatments. Some initial descriptions of "refrigerator mothers" as the cause has been long since dispelled. A neurological insult of multiple etiologies (genetic, intrauterine, neurotransmitter, or neurophysiological abnormalities) is posited. Parenting patterns do not cause autism. However, high parental skill level in working with his/her child may improve prognosis.

Although many children with more severe forms of ASD may be identified early, I find that schools commonly request consultation for children with mild "spectrum" disorders in the early elementary years. These children often present with tantrums as a key concern. The demands of school (for socially appropriate and conforming behavior) and the exquisite sensitivity of an ASD child to overstimulation, poor social and coping skills, and extreme need for sameness may overwhelm these youngsters. Oppositionality, obsessive-compulsive behaviors, and behavioral outbursts may be the primary complaint. A full evaluation followed by recommendations that allow the child to feel comfortable and not overwhelmed in the educational setting is often crucial to the child's ability to learn and the school's ability to provide for him or her.

Diagnostic Criterion and Epidemiology

It is estimated that 1% of the population may have a diagnosable autistic spectrum disorder. The number of children diagnosed with ASD has increased rapidly in the last 10 years, probably due to increased rate of detection of milder forms of the disorder, as well as potentially genetic or environmental contributors. The prevalence is greater in boys (except for Rett disorder). Girls with the disorder tend to be more severely affected. ASDs present in equal prevalence across race, ethnicity, and nationality. Table 5.1 summarizes the diagnostic criteria and epidemiology of the PDDs. Tables 5.2 and 5.3 summarize the etiology and differential diagnosis.

Comorbid Mental Disorders

Comorbidity is common with the ASDs. It is estimated that up to 80% of children with autism also have mental retardation. Anxiety disorders, obsessive-compulsive disorder, and

TABLE 5.1. Characteristics of the Pervasive Developmental Disorders

Disorder	Prevalence	Clinical Findings	Clinical Course
Autism	2–15 per 10,000 Boys, 4; Girls, 1 Girls generally with more severe disorder	Severe impairment of social interaction and communication Restricted, repetitive, and stereotypic patterns of behavior, interest, and activities Onset before age 3 Mental retardation common	Lifelong course Language skills and overall IQ are strongest prognostic indicators 25% have seizures in adolescence
Asperger disorder	Estimated 10–36 per 10,000 Boys, 5; Girls, 1	Impairment in social interactions Preoccupation with one or more restricted patterns of interest No delay in language or cognitive development Nonverbal learning disability cognitive profile common Motor clumsiness	Lifelong course Seem to improve as they mature Superior IQ improves prognosis 1/3 develop comorbid psychiatric disorders

Childhood disintegrative disorder	Estimated at 0.11 per 10,000 Boys, 8; Girls, 1	Normal development for at least 2 years Severe loss of developmental skills before 10 years of age	Skill loss usually occurs over a 6–9 month period, then plateaus Poor prognosis Mental retardation
Rett disorder	0.44 to 2.1 per 10,000 Girls only (rare reports of boys)	Normal at birth, but onset by 2 years Deceleration of head growth Loss of motor skills with hand-wringing movements; gait disturbance Loss of language Loss of social engagement	Severe regression in skills by age 2 Physically and socially debilitating High mortality (1.2%/yr)
PDD, NOS	2–16 per 10,000 Boys > Girls	"Atypical autism" Does not meet criteria for autism because of late age of onset, atypical symptoms, or subthreshold symptoms	Lifelong, but variable outcome Frequent comorbid psychiatric disorders

attention deficit hyperactivity disorder are all quite common. Tic disorders and psychotic symptoms are also notable comorbidities. Of note, a number of chromosomal disorders (especially fragile X and tuberous sclerosis) present with autistic-like features. Intrauterine viral infections, phenylkenouria, and seizure disorders are also associated. Table 5.4 summarizes components of a thorough evaluation.

 TIP

When you sit with a child, try to imagine the world through the child's eyes. If you find yourself feeling frustrated by your inability to engage the child, ignored or used as a tool, or having a very difficult time helping the child with a transition or reciprocal play, consider an ASD. More subtle forms of Asperger disorder may present in a very bright and interesting child who spends a session telling you about the details of his Yu-Gi-Oh cards (or any other area of fascination). It is the lack of flexibility, pedantic or professor-like speech, one-way nature of the communication, and high level of persistence in the topic that distinguish the child with mild Asperger disorder from a child who loves a hobby. Adults may delight in learning about the topic. Peers typically do not.

Treatment

Early detection and developmentally sensitive multimodal treatment are required for optimal outcomes. The primary intervention for ASDs is educational. Another key element is parent guidance and support, as this disorder is quite devastating to parents and families. Public Law 94-142, the Individuals with Disabilities Educational Act (IDEA), stipulates that every child, regardless of his or her disability, has a right to a free and appropriate public education in the least restrictive environment. For the eligible child, public educational services are mandated to begin at age 3. Key elements of early interventions include: 1) teaching the child to pay attention to other people, imitate others, use preverbal and verbal communication, play and socially interact; 2) a teaching environment that is highly supportive of the child's learning needs and involves systematic teaching of skills in a one-to-one setting with trained personnel; 3) a program that is predictable and routine; 4) a functional approach to problem behaviors; 5) a thoughtful strategy

TABLE 5.2. Etiology of Autism Spectrum Disorders

Type	Description
Hereditary	Multiple genes involved 50 times more prevalent in siblings High concordance (60–90%) in monozygotic twins Associated with other known genetic syndromes (e.g., fragile X and tuberous sclerosis)
Early alterations in embryonic development	Prenatal damage due to infection, toxins, and substance abuse, or etiology unknown
Neuroimaging findings	Ventricular enlargement/abnormal symmetry Cerebellum with hypoplasia Increased serotonin synthesis in dentate nucleus Lack of activation of fusiform gyrus (brain area that recognizes faces) Larger brains than typically developing children
Neurotransmitter abnormalities	Abnormalities in glutamate, serotonin, dopamine, opioid, and GABA neurotransmitters Autoimmune disorders/antibodies to serotonin-1A receptors

TABLE 5.3. Differential Diagnosis for Autism Spectrum Disorders

Disorder	Differentiating Features
Selective mutism	Child is able to speak and does so with family History of normal relatedness with family
Developmental language disorders	May use nonverbal cues; generally well related
Verbal apraxia/dyspraxias	Communicates nonverbally
Reactive attachment disorder	History of severe abuse/neglect
Attention deficit hyperactivity disorder	Able to make friends, even if their behavior makes sustaining friendships difficult
Mental retardation	Eye contact and relatedness spared
Childhood schizophrenia	Bizarre or unusual thoughts, hallucinations, loss of reality testing

TABLE 5.4. Evaluation Essentials for Children with Autism Spectrum Disorders

- Clinical History—focus on pre- and perinatal history, early social and language development, sensory sensitivities (to sounds, light, tactile stimulation, smells), odd or repetitive behaviors, ability to make transitions and changes in routine, family history, medical history.
- Evaluation of the child—focus on eye contact, ability to relate, ability for reciprocal and imaginative play or talk, note perseveration on a topic or activity, tone of voice and intonation, unusual movements or stereotypies, delayed or unusual speech, need for doing things in a particular manner or to be in charge of how things are done in a persistent and intense manner. Observation of the child's functioning in school or at home may also be helpful.
- Medical and neurological assessment and hearing evaluation (may require brainstem audiometry if child is not able to fully cooperate).
- Psychological testing to determine cognitive level, adaptive functioning scales (needed to diagnose mental retardation), academic testing to rule out learning disabilities and assist in academic planning. Speech and language testing, hearing testing, and occupational therapy and physical therapy evaluations should be completed as appropriate for the child. A young child should receive a developmental evaluation.
- Diagnostic scales: Autism Diagnostic Observation Schedule (ADOS) and Autism Diagnostic Intervien (ADI-R).

for transitioning from a specialized preschool classroom to the kindergarten class; 6) family involvement.

Treatment is multidisciplinary (teachers, mental health professionals, medical professionals, speech and language, occupational, and physical therapists, parents) and multimodal (utilization of multiple approaches targets the specific areas of disability, such as social, cognitive, motor, and academic). Table 5.5 summarizes the common educational, psychosocial, and pharmacological treatments used in providing for the complex child with ASD.

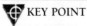 **KEY POINT**

Despite considerable attention in the lay press, there is no evidence that links the mumps, measles, and rubella (MMR) vaccine to autism. Due to the severity and chronicity of the disorder, a plethora of nonproven therapies have gained attention.

Many families will ask about these. They include nutritional supplements, elimination diets to combat food allergies, infusions of immune globulins, secretin, chelation therapy to remove mercury, facilitated communication (support of child's arm and hand while typing on keyboard), and others. There is lack of empiric support for all of these therapies, and education of families about the data and research is an important component of treatment.

CLINICAL VIGNETTE

Bob presented at age 3 with multiple problems including decreased and unusual language (echolalia, pronoun reversal), play which included lining up cars in pristine rows or spinning the wheels, and sensory sensitivities (tactile and loud noises). Bob's mother noted that his new 5-month-old sister smiles and looks at her more than Bob ever did. She assumed that Bob's difficulties had been due to his recurrent ear infections and lack of hearing. You refer for hearing testing, routine medical and neurological examinations, and developmental testing. Language and social skills deficits are notable, and you diagnose autism. Bob is enrolled in a preschool program, then half-day kindergarten. You consult again when he is 6 years old and in first grade.

Bob is very difficult to manage at school and at home. Bob throws tantrums for 1 to 2 hours if not allowed to do as he pleases. He is very active, inattentive, and does not sit still in school. The parents, initially resistant to medications, requested a medication assessment due to Bob's inability to comply with even simple commands and his lack of educational progress. A low dose of the stimulant methylphenidate was initiated for treatment of attention deficit hyperactivity symptoms. However, Bob demonstrated increased irritability and sleep disturbance with even very low doses of methylphenidate. Thus, it was discontinued, and a trial of the atypical antipsychotic risperidone was initiated for treatment of his inflexibility and agitation. Bob's motor activity decreased to a more age-appropriate level, tantrums decreased dramatically, and he was amenable to the school curriculum. In fact, the family was able to take a vacation together and enjoy it for the first time, with only minor outbursts by Bob.

TABLE 5.5. Treatment Essentials for Children with Autism Spectrum Disorders

Educational Approach	Comments	Reference
Applied behavioral analysis (ABA)	Plan that teaches appropriate behaviors that are to be generalized to all domains of a child's environment	Rosenwasser and Axelrod; Lovaas
Discrete trial training (DTT)	Teaching skills in specific situations	Grindle and Remington
Structured teaching	A system for organizing the environment and optimal conditions under which the child should be taught	Schopler
Developmental individual difference relationship model (DIR)	"Floortime"—uses relationship method to help the child relate and attend to the social setting	Greenspan and Wieder
Treatment and education of autistic and communication-handicapped children	Collaboration between mental health and educational professionals with parents to formulate an effective education and treatment plan	Schopler
Social stories	The use of stories to problem solve social dilemmas	Gray and Garand

Psychosocial Approach	Comments
Family support	Support groups, individual supportive counseling
Parent psychoeducation	Teaching parents about the disorder and collaboration in treatment planning
Parent behavioral management training	Use of behavioral specialist to help parents learn to employ behavior management protocols to help their child learn appropriate behavior
Public education system	Special educational services individualized to the needs of the child
Referral for special therapies (speech, occupational, physical)	Speech therapy for delays and to teach social speech OT for sensory processing and fine motor deficits PT for coordination deficits
Referral for disability services and support	Ensure that the child and family gain appropriate entitlements commensurate with the child and family's needs

Psychopharmacological Interventions	Target Symptoms	Comments
Antipsychotics: risperidone, olanzapine, quetiapine, aripiprazole, ziprasidone, haloperidol, thioridazine	Aggression, agitation, irritability, hyperactivity, and self-injurious behavior	The primary medications used to treat behavioral disturbances in ASD Most common adverse effects are weight gain, hyperlipidemia, hypertension, and increased prolactin

(Continued)

TABLE 5.5. Treatment Essentials for Children with Autism Spectrum Disorders (*continued*)

Psychopharmacological Interventions	Target Symptoms	Comments
SSRIs: fluoxetine, sertraline, citalopram, escitalopram, fluvoxamine	Anxiety, perseveration, compulsions, depression, and social isolation	Positive response may be correlated with family history of affective disorder Potential adverse effects are restlessness, insomnia, mania
Stimulants: methylphenidate, dextroamphetamines, amphetamine salts	Hyperactivity and inattention	Variable response More positive response with Asperger disorder May increase agitation and stereotypic behaviors
Alpha-2 agonists: guanfacine, clonidine	Hyperactivity, aggression, and sleep dysregulation	Clonidine is the more sedating
Anticonvulsants and lithium	Aggression and self-injurious behavior (SIB)	Need for blood monitoring may limit use May help mood lability
Naltrexone	Self-injurious behavior (SIB)	May be useful, but not robust data Need hepatic monitoring
Amantadine	Hyperactivity, irritability, and aggression	Need more studies
Melatonin	Sleep dysregulation	May be first line for insomnia

Disruptive Behavior Disorders

. . . .

6

Attention Deficit
Hyperactivity Disorder

Essential Concepts
- ADHD is a clinical diagnosis based on careful history taking, clinical examination, and information from multiple sources and multiple settings (school, home, community).
- The clinician must differentiate the core symptoms of ADHD from the secondary effects of other psychiatric disorders.
- Hyperactivity does not need to be present during the mental status exam to make the diagnosis of ADHD.
- Concomitant learning disabilities and comorbid psychiatric disorders should be evaluated.
- Baseline and follow-up rating scales are helpful in monitoring the effectiveness of treatment interventions and medication regimens.

Attention deficit hyperactivity disorder (ADHD) is the most commonly diagnosed psychiatric disorder of childhood and is characterized by deficits in attention, concentration, activity level, and impulse control. ADHD tends to run in families and is often associated with significant comorbidity with other psychiatric disorders, both externalizing (such as oppositional defiant disorder and conduct disorder) and internalizing (such as depression and anxiety), as well as bipolar disorder. The impact of ADHD on the child, his or her family, schools, and society is enormous, with billions of dollars spent annually for school services, mental health services, and increased use of the juvenile justice system. In contrast with historic notions, children do not typically "outgrow" ADHD. Morbidity and disability often persist into adult life. It is not infrequent that I have revealed the previously undiagnosed ADHD symptoms of a parent in the course of assessing his or her offspring. When his son was diagnosed with ADHD, one father exclaimed, "I am just like that—every little thing distracts me and I can't get my work done!" He was later evaluated and placed on a stimulant medication for ADHD, much to the benefit of his job effectiveness.

CLINICAL DESCRIPTION

The core symptoms needed to make a diagnosis of ADHD cover cognitive and/or motor symptoms grouped as inattention, and/or hyperactivity and impulsivity (Table 6.1).

TABLE 6.1. Diagnosis of ADHD

Inattentive Symptoms

When the child is inattentive, **CALL FOR FrEd.** This is a mnemonic to recall the nine criteria for the **Inattentive** symptoms of ADHD (6 of 9).

Careless mistakes
Attention difficulty
Listening problem
Loses things
Fails to finish what he/she starts
Organizational skills lacking
Reluctant to do tasks that require sustained mental effort
Forgetful in **R**outine activities
Easily **D**istracted

Hyperactive-Impulsive Symptoms

With hyperactivity-impulsive symptoms the child **RUNS FASTT.** This mnemonic covers the nine criteria for hyperactivity and inattention (6 of 9).

Runs or is restless
Unable to wait for his/her turn
Not able to play quietly
Slow—oh no, on the go
Fidgets with hands or feet
Answers are blurted out
Staying seated is difficult
Talks excessively
Tends to interrupt

Adapted from American Psychiatric Association (2000), Diagnostic and Statistical Manual of Mental Disorders, 4th ed. Text revision. Washington, DC. American Psychiatric Association.

The onset of ADHD impairment must be in early childhood, at least before the age of 7, even if it was not diagnosed until later in life. Additionally, the symptoms must be functionally impairing and present in a variety of life settings (home, school, work, etc.). ADHD should not be diagnosed if it presents only concomitantly with a pervasive developmental disorder or psychotic disorder, or if symptoms are likely a manifestation of another psychiatric disorder. If a child presents with 6 months of six or more of the inattentive symptoms, the disorder is identified as ADHD, Predominantly Inattentive Type. If there are 6 months of six or more hyperactive-impulsive symptoms, the criteria for Predominantly Hyperactive-Impulsive Type are met. If there are both, it is Combined Type.

 KEY POINT

Historically, the concept of ADHD has changed dramatically since its original description by Still in 1902 as a "morbid defect of moral control." Views of the disorder have been dominated by 1) behavior (e.g., hyperactivity); 2) etiology (e.g., minimal brain dysfunction); 3) and cognition (e.g. attention deficit disorder). The fluctuations in conceptualization over time have led to changes in diagnostic criteria, research designs, epidemiologic prevalence rates, and treatment interventions.

TIP

Don't rule out ADHD just because a child is able to attend and focus in your office one-on-one in an interesting activity or game. Many children with ADHD are able to sit still and pay attention in a highly structured or novel setting, when they are alone with an interested adult doing something they enjoy, or when engaged in a highly stimulating activity (such as videogames). Many ADHD children are able to attend to videogames for long periods of time. Symptoms typically worsen in situations that are unstructured, boring, or that require sustained attention or mental effort in a minimally stimulating venue (e.g., school work).

Epidemiology

ADHD is relatively common, affecting an estimated 3 to 12% of school-aged children, depending on the definition and study.

Epidemiological estimates have increased with DSM-IV classification of ADHD into three subtypes (inattentive, hyperactive-impulsive, and combined). In community samples of children, boys are diagnosed with ADHD-Combined Type at a frequency of 3:1 as compared to girls. Clinic samples tend to be 9:1 boys to girls, most likely due to the higher proportion of disruptive boys with ADHD-Combined Type, which may promote referral for treatment. Up to half of all children referred for mental health services are diagnosed with ADHD. The Inattentive Type of ADHD is not associated with an increase in disruptive behaviors and is more nearly equal in prevalence between boys and girls. This type is probably markedly underdiagnosed, as many of these children may be described as "dreamy," "slow," or "lazy," with lack of appreciation for the core inattentive symptoms.

 KEY POINT

ADHD is a disorder with major public health ramifications. Children have a higher injury rate, an increased risk for conduct disorder (one-third), criminal behavior, substance abuse, coordination deficits, and other psychiatric disorders (over half). There is an increased risk of physical punishments and abuse, and more stress within the family. Additionally, there is the economic cost to schools (over $3 billion/year), criminal justice system, health care system, social service agencies, and an increased risk for removal from the home.

Etiology

The etiology of ADHD remains unclear. However, it is certainly both multidetermined and complex. A mnemonic to remember the complex etiology is **GET TOPPS.**

Genetic—runs in families, but genetics not clear and likely polygenic; also fragile X, phenylketonuria, glucose-6-phosphate dehydrogenase deficiency correlated
Environmental—malnutrition, severe abuse and neglect in infancy
Toxic—lead or other poisoning
Trauma—head trauma
Other psychiatric disorders with comorbidity
Prenatal—maternal use of substances, poor health, very young mother, viral illness

Perinatal—low birth weight, hypoxia, prolonged labor, postmaturity, CNS infection

Subtle neurological deficits—smaller frontal lobe and hypoperfusion, asymmetry of the caudate nucleus, and smaller volume of cerebellar vermis

ADHD is a heterogeneous syndrome, with multifactorial etiology. Relative dysfunction of the prefrontal cortex, with subsequent deficits in "executive function" (planning, organization, and impulse control) is a common feature. Genetic determinants are suggested by family studies—up to one-third of children diagnosed with ADHD will have parents with ADHD. ADHD is two to three times more common in siblings. Candidate genes within the dopamine system are suspected, although genetics is most certainly complex, with the likelihood of multiple microchromosomal alterations leading to a similar phenotype (inattention). Fragile X and other specific genetic syndromes are associated with ADHD as well. Child-rearing practices do not cause ADHD. However, it is suspected that a severely chaotic early environment may adversely affect neuronal pruning and central nervous system (CNS) maturation. Any insult to the brain that results in subtle neurological deficits (hypoxia, head trauma, CNS infections, and suboptimal pre- and perinatal conditions) may predispose to ADHD. Imaging findings are not specific enough to be used for diagnosis. However, there is a correlation with smaller and hypoperfused frontal lobes, asymmetry of the caudate nucleus, and smaller cerebellar vermis. Functional magnetic resonance imaging (fMRI) research may more clearly elucidate some of the subtle neurological deficits associated with difficulties with attention and impulse control.

Assessment

ADHD is a clinical diagnosis made on the basis of interviews and rating scales. There is no specific laboratory or other test. The assessment of ADHD is similar to a full psychiatric evaluation for any other disorder. It may be tempting to merely start a stimulant medication to "see if it helps." However, knowing family history and ruling out other primary or comorbid psychiatric disorders, medical problems, substance abuse, or side effects of other medications are critical. Talking to school personnel about the key difficulties in school and assessing functional disability in multiple domains are also key.

Children and adolescents with ADHD commonly are less aware than others around them of their maladaptive symptoms. The patient may deny symptoms entirely, so the diagnosis cannot be based on patient report. However, meeting with the child is essential. Observation in the school setting may be most useful. Meeting the child and completing a child interview and mental status examination and a medical screening (neurological soft signs, tics and coordination difficulties, height, weight, blood pressure, and pulse) are routine. Lab work to rule out lead exposure, thyroid problems, or other medical difficulties may be obtained, as appropriate. Ensuring that hearing and vision are normal is also needed. Psychological testing is useful to assess intellectual ability, academic achievement, and possible specific learning disorders. ADHD is frequently comorbid with learning disorders, but the oppositionality and inattention that may be precipitated by learning difficulties need to be clarified. Neuropsychological testing can clarify deficits in executive functioning and sustained attention, and the Continuous Performance Test (a computerized test of distractibility and attention) may be helpful. However, all tests are useful in the context of a full evaluation, and none is diagnostic in and of itself.

🜨 KEY POINT

Obtaining information from multiple informants is critical to the diagnosis of ADHD—especially school personnel (ask about learning, attentional issues, and behavioral problems), as well as the primary care physician (for birth and medical history) and parents (prenatal and perinatal history, medical history, screening questions for sleep disorders, traumatic events, the potential for lead poisoning, family psychiatric and medical history). I recommend using an ADHD rating scale (parent and teacher forms) for both diagnosis and follow-up of treatment effectiveness.

Comorbidity and Differential Diagnosis

Individuals with ADHD are at increased risk of suffering from other psychiatric disorders. The most common comorbidities are summarized in Table 6.2.

It is important to diagnose comorbid disorders since the ADHD child with another psychiatric condition may have a

TABLE 6.2. Common Comorbid Disorders Associated with Attention Deficit Hyperactivity Disorder

Disorder	Estimated % Associated with ADHD[a]
Oppositional defiant disorder or conduct disorder	50%
Learning disabilities	40% (20%–60%)
Anxiety disorder	30% (25%–33%)
Major depression	30% (3%–75%)
Bipolar disorder	10%–20% of clinical samples

[a]ADHD, attention deficit hyperactivity disorder.

different clinical presentation, life course, and response to treatment. The most common comorbidities with ADHD are disruptive behavior disorders, mood disorders (bipolar disorder and major depressive disorder), and anxiety disorders.

ADHD must be differentiated from age-appropriate over-activity and other disorders. The differential diagnosis for ADHD is extensive, as summarized in Table 6.3.

Treatment

ADHD is a complex disorder affecting every area of functioning and thereby requires a comprehensive treatment program. The essentials of an effective treatment plan include psychosocial interventions, medication treatment, and ensuring an appropriate educational plan (Table 6.4).

As highlighted in the large multimodal treatment of ADHD (MTA) study, medication is the most effective treatment for the core symptoms of ADHD. There is a large body of literature documenting the efficacy of stimulants on core features of ADHD (motoric overactivity, impulsivity, and inattentiveness) as well as substantial effects on cognition, social function, and aggression. The stimulant medications are the best-studied medications in child and adolescent psychiatry and have demonstrated safety and efficacy in over 200 controlled studies. Concern about cardiovascular effects, especially blood pressure and pulse (particularly for Adderal XR), has prompted increased scrutiny around the safety of the stimulant medications by the U.S. Food and Drug Administration. Despite concerns of many families about the abuse potential of the medication and the risk of precipitating addiction, treatment with stimulant medication

TABLE 6.3. Essential Differential Diagnosis for Attention Deficit Hyperactivity Disorder

Psychiatric disorders
Oppositional defiant disorder
Conduct disorder
Mood disorders (depression and bipolar disorder)
Anxiety disorders
Tic disorders
Substance use disorders
Pervasive developmental disorder
Learning disorders
Posttraumatic stress disorder
Mental retardation or borderline intellectual functioning
Psychosocial conditions
Abuse and/or neglect
Poor nutrition
Neighborhood violence
Chaotic family situation
Being bullied at school
Medical disorders
Partial deafness or poor eyesight
Seizure disorder
Fetal alcohol syndrome/effects
Genetic abnormalities (such as fragile X)
Sedating or activating medications
Thyroid abnormality
Heavy metal poisoning

has actually been demonstrated to decrease the risk for substance abuse, legal difficulties, and other sequelae of poor impulse control.

There are several treatment options for ADHD tailored to patient need. In general, stimulant medications are considered first line in the treatment of the core symptoms of ADHD. Common side effects include loss of appetite, sleep disturbance, and some changes in pulse and blood pressure. More serious side effects include dysphoria, irritability, and the potential precipitation or exacerbation of tics.

Several antidepressants have been used as second line for ADHD, with atomoxetine (Straterra) being FDA approved for this indication. However, the "black box" warning of an increased risk for suicidal thoughts and behavior for antidepressant use in children and adolescents also applies to atomoxetine.

TABLE 6.4. Essentials of Treatment for ADHD

Psychosocial Treatments

Parent psychoeducation—education about the disorder, teaching how to manage the environment to assist the child (consistency, routines, organization, reducing stimulation, decreasing frustration and anticipating difficulties, behavior management)

Psychotherapy—social skills training, cognitive-behavior therapy (to learn social and academic problem-solving strategies and ability to manage frustration), and behavior modification; individual psychotherapy may be useful in addressing comorbid disorders, issues of self-esteem, or sequelae of trauma

Group therapy—to help the child gain social skills

Family psychotherapy/Parent management training—to reduce conflict and improve communication and problem solving within the family

Educational/School-Related Interventions

Psychoeducational assessment (cognitive and behavioral assessment, ADHD rating scales, etc.)

Teacher and classroom modifications—teacher understanding the disorder and appropriate classroom modifications [preferential seating of child near teacher; consistent classroom structure and routines; organizational skills teaching such as schedule, assisting child in organizing notebooks and materials, assignment and homework notebook; cuing plan for teacher to cue child to attend without calling negative attention to the child; extra supervision in unstructured activities (lunch, recess, etc.); behavioral management plan (may include Daily Report Card which targets specific behaviors to be shared between home and school); social skills group]

Special education or Section 504 services—provides extra supports for children whose ADHD is interfering with educational progress. A small, self-contained classroom or resource room, one-to-one tutoring, or a more intensive therapeutic educational plan or out-of-district special education placement for severely disruptive behaviors may be required

Medication Treatment

Considered first line
Methylphenidate: Ritalin,[a] Ritalin SR,[a] Concerta,[a] Metadate,[a] Focalin[a]
Dextroamphetamine: Dexedrine,[a] Dextrostat[a]
Amphetamine salts: Adderall[a]

Second line
Atomoxetine (Straterra)[a,b]
Bupropion (Wellbutrin)[b]   ↑ suicidality risk
Venlafaxine (Effexor)[b]

(Continued)

TABLE 6.4. Essentials of Treatment for ADHD (*continued*)

Medication Treatment

TCAs: nortriptyline, desipramine, imipramine[b]

Guanfacine (Tenex)—alpha agonist, most useful for hyperactivity and overarousal

Clonidine (Catapres)—alpha agonist, may be first line for child with ADHD and tics

Modafinil (Provigil, Cephalon)—used for narcolepsy and preliminary studies for ADHD

Considered when most other medications are ineffective

Atypical antipsychotics: risperidone, olanzapine, quetiapine, ziprasidone—most helpful in treating agitation and aggression

Typical antipsychotics: haloperidol,[a] thioridazine,[a] chlorpromazine (Thorazine)

MAOIs: phenelzine, tranylcypromine, selegine—not generally used because of food restrictions

Pemoline (Cylert)[a,c]—may cause liver toxicity

TCAs, tricyclic antidepressants; MAOIs, monoamine oxidase inhibitors.

[a]U.S. Food and Drug Administration (FDA)-approved for treatment of ADHD.

[b]Black box warning for increased risk of suicidality.

[c]Black box warning for hepatotoxicity.

 TIP

Consider clonidine first line for the treatment of ADHD with moderate tics. For children and adolescents with a pervasive developmental disorder that includes functionally impairing ADHD symptoms, start very low on stimulant dosage, due to increased risk of irritability and stereotypies.

CLINICAL VIGNETTE

Kate is a 10-year-old fifth-grade girl who is referred for treatment of difficulties with anxiety and oppositionality. She has a history of separation anxiety in kindergarten and is described as sensitive and kind. She is getting Ds and Fs in several of her academic classes due to failure to complete assignments. She avoids written schoolwork and tends to be oppositional (needs at least three prompts to follow through with directions). The teacher feels that Kate is quite preoccupied, doesn't listen, is "dreamy" (perhaps worrying?), and is not available for learning. You take a full history and discover that Kate had low normal developmental milestones. She is more dependent on her mother than most other children her age and more than her brother 2 years her junior. Her mother complains that her room is a disorganized mess, and that it is "like pulling teeth" to get Kate to get ready for school or any activity in the morning. It is as if she is in slow motion. She often forgets instructions and seems easily distracted. She tends to take a very long time to complete any assignment, and avoids school work. Her writing is slow and labored. You request psychological testing, which suggests average cognitive functioning and no specific learning disability, with some delays in processing speed and executive functioning. An ADHD scale is positive for inattentive symptoms, but not hyperactivity or impulsivity. Anxiety level is higher than in most children, but there are no acute worries. Sleep and appetite are normal. You diagnose ADHD, inattentive type, and wonder about a comorbid anxiety disorder. You begin a low-dose stimulant (methylphenidate, 5 mg) and increase slowly. Within a few weeks Kate is getting her classwork completed for the first time in her life. Her grades improve and oppositionality decreases—she is less work avoidant. You switch to a long-acting preparation, as Kate does not want to go to the nurse during the school day (Concerta, 18 mg and increased to 36 mg over time). Her teacher notes a dramatic improvement in Kate's school functioning. Additionally, upon your recommendation, Kate's seat is placed closer to the teacher, she gets extra time for tests and can take tests in a quiet area, and the teacher has found a nonintrusive manner to prompt Kate to pay attention. Kate and her teacher have worked out a checklist for organization of her materials and a homework log. If Kate misses a morning dosage of medication, both she and her teacher can note the difference. Kate did not demonstrate an increase in anxiety symptoms.

 TIP

Not all children with ADHD are hyperactive. The inattentive type may present with slow processing and a sluggish cognitive and behavioral style which suggests dreaminess, disinterest, or oppositionality and avoidance (not following directions). This subtype may be particularly responsive to stimulant medication.

Prognosis

About three-quarters of children diagnosed with ADHD continue to show symptoms of ADHD into adolescence, and conduct difficulties are common (about one-third of children with ADHD).

Follow-up studies into adulthood show that up to half of individuals diagnosed with ADHD continue to suffer from clinically significant symptoms. Furthermore, up to 33% of ADHD individuals versus less than 10% of controls drop out of high school. ADHD children often show secondary effects such as low self-esteem and poor social skills. These individuals tend to obtain less education overall by 2 to 3 years and lower occupational rankings, and have more car accidents, court appearances and convictions, suicide attempts, and problems with relationships than do young adults without ADHD. Children with ADHD with conduct disorder are also at increased risk for developing substance use disorders and antisocial personality in adulthood.

Despite this seemingly grim prognosis, many children with ADHD become well-adjusted, high-achieving adults. Prognosis is improved with effective treatment, appropriate educational programming, high cognitive, athletic, and interpersonal abilities, and an emotionally supportive family with adequate social and financial resources.

Conduct Disorder and Oppositional Defiant Disorder

Essential Concepts

- A behavior disorder must be differentiated from normal oppositionality as a child gains more autonomy, a consequence of another disorder, or a comorbid disorder.
- ODD and CD are clinical diagnoses based on careful history taking, clinical examination, and information from multiple sources and multiple settings (school, home, community).
- Concomitant learning disabilities and comorbid psychiatric disorders should be evaluated.
- There are evidence-based psychosocial treatments for CD that should be utilized.

The disruptive behavior disorders (also sometimes called "externalizing disorders") include oppositional defiant disorder (ODD), conduct disorder (CD), and attention deficit hyperactivity disorder (ADHD). ODD and CD are closely related, with ODD being viewed as a precursor, milder form, or subtype of CD. These disorders characterize children and adolescents whose behaviors reflect social rule violations and inappropriate actions against others. Often the behaviors are much more upsetting to those around them than to the child or adolescent that is displaying the behaviors. It is important to note that many preadolescents and adolescents are oppositional, and this, in and of itself, is not considered a disorder. It is when the behaviors occur much more frequently than is typically observed with individuals of comparable age and developmental level and when it is functionally impairing that it becomes a disorder. I also find it essential to thoroughly investigate for other primary disorders or comorbidities. Many traumatized, mood disordered (depressed or bipolar), psychotic, or developmentally disabled youth will engage in very bad behaviors. ODD or CD should not be diagnosed separately if symptoms occur exclusively during the course of these other disorders.

The disruptive behavior disorders are a serious public health problem in the United States. Conduct symptoms are the reason for inpatient and outpatient psychiatric treatment of one-third to one-half of youth using these services. CD has been identified as the most costly mental health problem in the United States. Children with serious conduct symptoms are likely to become involved in multiple services systems (e.g., mental health, juvenile justice, special education), and this may continue throughout childhood and well into adulthood.

CLINICAL DESCRIPTION

Table 7.1 summarizes the diagnostic criteria for ODD and CD.

There must be at least three symptoms within the past year, and at least one of the symptoms evident in the last 6 months to make a CD diagnosis. The symptoms must be repetitive, persistent, functionally impairing, and present in a variety of life settings (home, school, work, etc.). If the individual is 18 years or older, he or she does not meet criteria for antisocial personality disorder. Conduct disorder is subdivided by age of onset (childhood onset with at least one criterion before the age of 10; adolescent onset with no symptoms prior to the age of 10; unspecified onset when the age of onset is not known).

✦ KEY POINT

Although usually conduct disorder is considered "externalizing," in that the behavior violates others, it is also strongly associated with aggression toward the self. Adolescents with concomitant depression, conduct disorder, and substance abuse are at a substantially higher risk for suicide. This is true for males and females. However, males tend to use more lethal methods. The potential for suicide should be routinely assessed with conduct-disordered youth.

⚡ TIP

Many children and youth with ODD and CD are able to behave appropriately when highly motivated. An interview with a charming and engaged adolescent does not rule out the possibility of significant conduct issues. As many youth with disruptive disorders do not conceptualize their behaviors as problematic (and may either minimize or lie about them), a full evaluation with multiple informants is required.

TABLE 7.1. Diagnostic Criteria of ODD and CD

Oppositional Defiant Disorder

When children and adolescents are oppositional and defiant they act like **REAL BADS.** For ODD, the individual must show at least four of eight symptoms within the past 6 months. This is a mnemonic to recall the criteria for the oppositional defiant disorder:

Resentful
Easily annoyed
Argues with adults
Loses temper
Blames others for his or her misbehavior
Annoys people deliberately
Defies rules or requests
Spiteful

Conduct Disorder

The behaviors of Conduct Disorder are **BAD FOR A BUSINESS.** This mnemonic covers the criteria for conduct disorder (3 of 15 in past year and 1 in past 6 months):

Bullying
Animal cruelty
Destroying others' property
Fighting
Out late at night
Running away from home
Actively forcing sex
Being cruel to people
Using a weapon
Setting fires
Into someone's house, building, or car
Not going to school
Everyday lying or conning others
Stealing while confronting a victim
Stealing without confronting a victim

Adapted from American Psychiatric Association (2000), Diagnostic and Statistical Manual of Mental Disorders, 4th ed. Text revision. Washington, DC. American Psychiatric Association.

Epidemiology

Anywhere between 2 and 16% of school-aged children are believed to meet diagnostic criteria for ODD and/or CD. Both ODD and CD are more prevalent in boys than in girls. Rates of CD tend to be higher for adolescents (7% for youth ages 12–16) than for children (4% for children ages 4–11). Childhood-onset CD is considered to be a more serious form of the disorder and generally has a worse prognosis. Even so, less than half of conduct-disordered children continue to suffer from CD into adulthood. However, some type of psychiatric disorder is diagnosed in up to 80% of adults who had CD as children. In general, CD children grown up will demonstrate higher rates of criminality, psychiatric and substance abuse disorders, lower academic and occupational achievement, poorer marital and social relationships, and poorer physical health than their non-CD peers.

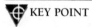 KEY POINT

Comorbidity and differential diagnosis are important to assess. Many psychiatric disorders are associated with behavioral symptoms, and "pure" CD without comorbidities is relatively rare. The most common comorbidities for CD are ADHD (about one third of ADHD children will have CD, and up to 70% of CD children will have ADHD). Other common comorbidities are anxiety disorders, bipolar disorder, depression, adjustment disorder, trauma-related disorders, and developmental disorders.

Etiology

The etiology of ODD and CD is complex and multifactorial. Research has focused on multiple risk factors that contribute to the onset. These factors are characteristics, events, or processes that increase the likelihood for the onset of the disorder (Table 7.2). However, children may have multiple risk factors and never have the disorder, or contrariwise, may have a few and exhibit the full disorder. Although much remains to be elucidated, a great deal is known about the onset of CD, and research will likely enable us to subdivide the disorder into types that may have unique etiologies and unique effective treatment methods (Table 7.3 and Table 7.4).

TABLE 7.2. Factors That Place Youth at Risk for ODD or CD

Child Factors

Temperament: child with more difficult temperament (negative mood, less adaptability, etc.) and high level of novelty seeking

Neuropsychological deficits: deficits in language functioning, memory, motor coordination, and "executive functioning" (e.g., abstract reasoning, planning, focused attention, and judgment)

Low autonomic activity/arousal

Early behavior difficulties: early onset of unmanageability and aggression

Academic difficulties: learning disorders and lower levels of intellectual functioning

Serotonergic dysfunction

Head injury, seizures, and other neurological insults

Other psychiatric disorders (esp. ADHD, PTSD, LDs, substance abuse, mood disorders)

Parent and Family Factors

Pre- and perinatal complications: pregnancy and birth complications, prematurity and low birth weight, minor birth injury or complications

Psychopathology and criminal behavior in the family: criminal behavior, antisocial personality, and alcoholism of a parent

Family history of antisocial personality, substance use, ADHD, mood disorder, LDs

Poor parenting: coercive parent–child communications, inconsistent discipline, harsh or physical punishment, and permissive or overcontrolling parent

Poor supervision: few rules and lack of supervision

Impaired quality of family relationships: less parental acceptance of their children, less warmth, affection, emotional support, and attachment

Marital discord: conflict and/or domestic violence

Family size: larger family size

Siblings with antisocial behavior (esp. older brother with antisocial behavior)

Socioeconomic disadvantage: poverty, overcrowding, unemployment, poor housing, financial stress and lack of supports

School-Related Factors

Inadequate school environment: large classroom with little emphasis on academics, infrequent teacher use of positive feedback, little emphasis on individual responsibility of students, poor facilities and work space, unavailability of teachers and other support staff to deal with student difficulties

(Continued)

TABLE 7.2. Factors That Place Youth at Risk for ODD or CD (*Continued*)

Protective Factors

Factors that decrease the probability of exhibiting CD among otherwise high risk youth: being first born, perceived by their mothers as affectionate, high self-esteem and locus of control (feel that their behavior can make a difference), and having adults who play an important role in their development (in addition to parents) who are supportive same-sex adult role models

Treatment

Treatment is most effective if it is multimodal, utilized in a variety of settings, and includes a home, school, and child component to the treatment. Conduct disorder has well-studied evidence-based psychosocial treatments that should be utilized. Early intervention and helping families gain more adaptive methods of relating improve prognosis (Table 7.4).

Prognosis

The prognosis for ODD and CD is quite variable. Many children with CD continue to demonstrate some fluctuating difficulties with behavioral issues on 7-year follow-up. About one-third of individuals with CD will develop antisocial personality disorder. Low IQ score and parental antisocial

TABLE 7.3. Essentials of Assessment of ODD and CD

1. Multimethod, multirater, and multisetting assessments should be made.
2. Rating scales may be helpful, but not diagnostic.
3. Ensure a complete psychiatric evaluation for other primary diagnoses or comorbidities.
4. An educational assessment should be performed if school or learning problems are suspected. Rule out learning disabilities, cognitive deficits, or sensory loss (hearing or vision problems).
5. Evaluate the family dynamics, interactions, and communication style, as well as family history of disorders.
6. Perform functional behavioral analysis of the behavior patterns, including antecedents, consequences, and baseline and follow-up ratings of behaviors.

TABLE 7.4. Treatment for Conduct Disorder

Evidence-based Psychosocial Treatments

Parent-management training (PMT)	Trains parents to interact with the child in ways that promote prosocial behavior
Cognitive problem-solving skills training	Develops skills in approaching interpersonal conflicts, reframing cognitive expectations, and practicing adaptive solutions
Multisystemic therapy	Focus on the family system functioning and the child's behavior within the context of multiple systems (family, school, peer group, etc.)
Anger-management training	Helps child develop more adaptive methods to cope with angry feelings
Functional family therapy	Focuses on helping the family improve interactional style and functional behaviors

Pharmacological Treatments

Therapeutic Class	Medication	Clinical Effect
Stimulants	Methylphenidate preparations	Dose-dependent
	Amphetamine salts	Reduce disinhibited behavior
Mood stabilizers	Lithium	Decrease behavioral dyscontrol
	Anticonvulsants	
Antipsychotics	Risperidone	Reduce level of CNS activation
	Clozapine	
	Chlorpromazine	
	Haloperidol	
	Droperidol	

(Continued)

TABLE 7.4. Treatment for Conduct Disorder *(Continued)*

Pharmacological Treatments

Adrenergic agents	Clonidine	Increase frustration tolerance
	Guanfacine	
	Propranolol	
	Pindolol	
	Nadolol	
	Metoprolol	

Other Interventions

Intensive community-based services
Therapeutic schools
Residential treatment

personality disorder predict persistence of CD. More positive outcome is predicted by a lower severity of CD, fewer ADHD symptoms, higher verbal IQ, greater family socioeconomic advantage, and biological parents who were not antisocial.

Prevention and early intervention tend to be most successful in improving prognosis. Despite the high risk for other psychiatric disorders, incarceration, and impairment in occupational functioning, many children with CD achieve a favorable adult adjustment.

CLINICAL VIGNETTE:

Joe is a 7-year-old boy who was raised in a single-parent home in a socioeconomically disadvantaged area. He is the third of four children. His mother is highly stressed, and his father is incarcerated for stealing a car (likely to support his substance habit). Joe was potentially exposed early in utero to cocaine and alcohol, although his mother stopped using substances when she found out that she was pregnant. You are asked to consult to the school because Joe is demonstrating severe behavioral issues at school. He gets into frequent fights with peers, threw a rock at another child after school, talks back and swears at the teachers, and refuses to do his work. He has teased and bullied other children. He recently was reported to have shown his buttocks and attempted to touch another boy's buttocks in the school restroom. What are the key components of the assessment you will need to help diagnose and set up a treatment plan for Joe?

 TIP

I suggest meeting with teachers, the mother, any social service agencies involved (which are likely given the child's possible touching of another child; find out the status of any present protective service investigations with informed consent), and the primary care physician to clarify developmental (including early neglect, sexual or physical abuse) and social history. Get more complete family history of psychiatric, substance abuse, and legal issues. In this case, psychological testing will be needed to ascertain cognitive functioning and potential learning disabilities. Tests for executive functioning should be included. The Behavior Assessment Scale for Children (BASC teacher and parent form) and an ADHD rating form may also be helpful. A class or recess observation is recommended. Interview the child and ask about abuse, neglect, psychotic symptoms, mood symptoms, anxiety symptoms, and safety issues. Ask about smoking or drugs. Ask the child to draw his family doing something together. Ask about the child's three wishes. Inquire about issues of guilt and remorse. Does the child have insight into how his behavior affects others? In this case, PTSD (neglect and sexual abuse by an older cousin when the child was 4), ADHD, and a reading disability were diagnosed. The conduct issues were assessed to emanate from these other disorders, and a separate CD diagnosis was not made at this time. However, treatment planning included interventions to address the severe behavioral issues.

PART C
Other Disorders of Infancy, Childhood, or Adolescence
. . . .

 Separation Anxiety Disorder

Essential Concepts
- Separation anxiety disorder (SAD) commonly presents with somatic symptoms such as stomachaches or headaches to avoid leaving home.
- About three-fourths of children with SAD exhibit school avoidance.
- Children with SAD experience unrealistic fears that they or their parents will be injured, kidnapped, or killed.
- Children with SAD are disabled by their inability to sleep alone, attend school, visit friends, or stay at camp.

Separation anxiety disorder (SAD) is a common disorder of children, and is characterized by extreme anxiety and worry concerning separation from home or from those to whom the individual is attached. It is often first diagnosed in preschool or kindergarten, when the child experiences a separation from home and the "attachment object." Although some anxiety symptoms may persist, separation anxiety disorder is generally a disorder of childhood, and remits with advancing age.

CLINICAL DESCRIPTION

Table 8.1 provides criteria for a diagnosis of SAD.

TABLE 8.1. Diagnosis of Separation Anxiety Disorder

When the child is frightened of being separated he or she will **PUSH** or **NAGS**. This is a mnemonic to recall the eight criteria for Separation Anxiety Disorder (three of eight required).

Physical symptoms and complaints with anticipated separation
Untoward event anxiety
Sleep difficulties
Harm to attachment figures a concern
Nightmares
Alone is a big fear
Going to school or out of home difficult
Separation fears

The onset of symptoms must be in childhood, occur for at least 4 weeks, and cause clinically significant impairment.

Adapted from American Psychiatric Association (2000), Diagnostic and Statistical Manual of Mental Disorders, 4th ed. Text revision. Washington, DC. American Psychiatric Association.

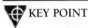 KEY POINT

In SAD, somatic symptoms such as headache, stomachache, nausea, and vomiting are common, and medical assessment should be done to rule out a primary medical etiology. However, in SAD the somatic symptoms are typically absent on weekends, holidays, and when there are no separations. The symptoms occur on evenings and mornings before school or before an anticipated separation.

 TIP

Children with separation anxiety will typically have a great deal of difficulty at the start of each school year. I recommend to families that the child have a structured out-of-home summer plan (usually a day camp) to decrease the regression that is typical when a child stays home with the attachment figure most of the summer. Additionally, I typically recommend supportive and anxiety management psychotherapy beginning several weeks prior to the start of school. Working with the school system to have a support system in place is also crucial. I suggest that the school social worker or psychologist form a strong relationship with the child, and meet the child at the beginning of the school day to help with the school transition. SAD is a disorder that needs strong collaboration between the therapist, school personnel, parents, and child to help decrease distress and disability.

Epidemiology

The prevalence of SAD is estimated to be 2.4 to 4.7% of the population of children. Males seem to be affected about equally to females.

Etiology

Anxiety disorders tend to aggregate in families. SAD is likely precipitated by the interaction of genetic, temperament, family dynamics, and other environmental factors. The temperamental construct of "behavioral inhibition to the unfamiliar" describes the shy, cautious, and introverted child. Children with this temperamental disposition may be at increased risk for SAD, as well as other anxiety disorders. Parents with anxiety disorders may provide genetic vulnerability, as well as unwittingly convey their own fearfulness, to which the child reacts with fearfulness as well.

Assessment

The assessment includes a standard complete psychiatric evaluation. Multiple informants (the primary care physician, school or preschool personnel, parents, etc.) are key. The assessment should focus on symptoms of anxiety and/or mood disorders in both the child and parents. A parent may need to be present for the entire interview of the child if he or she is unable to separate. The information gleaned from attempting a separation must be weighed against the trust and comfort of the child in the therapeutic relationship and his or her need for the parent to be present. Typically, history is sufficient for the diagnosis. The differential diagnosis includes other anxiety disorders, depressive disorders, as well as pervasive developmental disorders or psychosis.

Treatment

Treatment of SAD is multimodal, and includes psychosocial and school interventions. Additionally, medications may be indicated when the symptoms are severe and disabling.

The psychosocial interventions include cognitive-behavioral, individual educational/supportive, and/or psychodynamic psychotherapy combined with parent guidance, behavior modification, family therapy, and school consultation.

The child will benefit from learning relaxation skills. Sleep disturbance or resistance to sleeping alone typically responds positively to systematic monitoring of bedtime behavior, gradual weaning of parental presence (including sitting outside of the open door for a period of time), and relaxation skills. Psychodynamic psychotherapy may help children with SAD resolve conflicts and achieve mastery over separation and autonomy. Transference and working through separations with the therapist are key.

Parents must be involved in the therapy to reassure the child as he or she achieves more independence and autonomy. School interventions include working with the school personnel to support the child's school attendance, providing added support to the child in dealing with anxiety, and using relaxation and other techniques to help the child feel more comfortable at school. Appropriate limits around requested phone calls home and a plan for somatic symptoms and nurse visits should be anticipated. A behavioral plan with reinforcements for appropriate school behavior is recommended. At times, children may require a partial hospital program or modified school program to allow a transition to school reentry. Home-bound education is contraindicated.

Medication treatment is typically with the selective serotonin reuptake inhibitors (SSRIs) for treatment of anxiety with or without depression. Tricyclic antidepressants may also be considered. Benzodiazepines may be indicated for the acute treatment of school refusal—but treatment should be brief and focused, with monitoring for behavioral disinhibition.

◆ KEY POINT

School refusal may be considered a psychiatric urgency (not quite an emergency, but requiring prompt and intensive intervention). The longer the child is out of school, the greater the treatment resistance, chronicity, and school failure. If a child with SAD is refusing to go to school, an intensive treatment plan needs to be formulated quickly and collaboratively—to include family, school, and child components. Medication to help decrease the level of anxiety may be quite helpful. The temporary use of benzodiazepines may be indicated in this urgent clinical crisis.

Selective Mutism

9

> ### Essential Concepts
> - Selective mutism is a fairly rare disorder of childhood characterized by the ability to understand language and speak, but to do so only in certain situations.
> - This disorder is often very frustrating to teachers and parents, who are at a loss as to how to get the child to speak.
> - Children with selective mutism may have academic underachievement and impaired peer relationships due to their lack of speaking.

Selective mutism is a fascinating disorder of children who are able to speak, but refuse to do so in public situations. Child and adolescent psychiatrists are often consulted when the disorder has become more chronic and is interfering with educational and social adjustment. It is typically first diagnosed in preschool or kindergarten, when the child is first expected to interact in a broader social environment. There may be a link between selective mutism in children and social phobia in adults.

CLINICAL DESCRIPTION

A child with selective mutism consistently does not speak in specific social situations in which there is an expectation for speaking, such as school. The child is able to speak in other situations. The symptoms must persist for at least 1 month and be severe enough to negatively impact educational and interpersonal functioning.

Epidemiology

Selective mutism has a prevalence of less than 1% of school-age children in mental health settings (about 0.7% prevalence overall). Girls are thought to be affected twice as often as boys.

TIP

Children with selective mutism are typically extremely aware of the frustration they are causing to the adults and peers in the environment. They are also usually hypervigilant about covert attempts to "get them to talk." A referral to "get the child to talk" in school needs to be quickly reframed, as this type of control struggle rarely is effective and frequently exacerbates the disorder. Helping the child to feel comfortable, to participate, to make friends, and to be academically successful are more appropriate goals. The other children in the class need to be educated to minimize their concern about the selectively mute child speaking and not to overly react if the child does speak. I have seen children who are beginning to speak shut down again if their peers or teachers are too joyful about the utterances.

Etiology

Selective mutism is thought to be an anxiety disorder, possibly an early form of developing social phobia. Parents of selectively mute children have a higher incidence of anxiety disorders, such as panic, social and performance anxiety, and others. Biological factors such as genetic predisposition to anxiety disorders and temperament are thought to be contributory.

Selectively mute children often also have experienced developmental delays in speech and language. About half of these children have speech immaturities or a speech disorder. Nonspecific neurodevelopmental disorders are also more common.

Some children with selective mutism have a history of trauma. Abuse, early hospitalization, family instability, and frequent moves may also contribute to the development of symptoms in some children.

Assessment

The assessment includes a standard complete psychiatric evaluation. Neurological and hearing assessment, physical examination for oral-facial abnormalities, cognitive testing for mental retardation, and speech and language evaluation are generally indicated. Frequently, parents will need to describe speech patterns and developmental history in considerable detail, as the child rarely will speak to the examiner. Nonverbal tests of intelligence (such as the Leiter scale or TONI [Test of Nonverbal Intelligence]) may be required. Family patterns of communication should be investigated. Family history of anxiety disorder should be elicited. Although the child will likely not speak, assessment of drawings, play, and relatedness are important. Differential diagnosis includes communication and cognitive disorders, hearing loss, pervasive developmental disorders, psychotic disorders, and conversion disorder.

Therapy

Therapy of selective mutism is based on the assumption that the child will speak again if he or she feels safe and comfortable. Any form of communication is encouraged through behavioral plans that shape progressive communication, interventions to decrease anxiety, and the formation of trusting relationships. The overall philosophy is a nonconfrontational collaborative approach to helping the child gain more adaptive functioning. Behavior therapy and parent counseling tend to be more effective than individual psychotherapy. The identification and focus on secondary reinforcement and family patterns that maintain symptoms are crucial. Clear and nonconfrontational articulation by the parents, school personnel, and therapist of the expectation that the child communicate is important. It is not helpful to have a sibling or other routinely talk for the patient. Medications to treat the anxiety disorder are typically the SSRIs.

CLINICAL VIGNETTE

Jenny is a 6-year-old first-grade student about whom you are consulted because of concerns that she has never spoken at school, despite parental reassurance that she speaks at home. Jenny is a fraternal twin, and has been the shyer of the two. Her twin sister, a popular and social child, often speaks for Jenny.

Jenny has never spoken in school, although she will sometimes mouth the words without vocalization. Jenny does speak at home, and if children are visiting her home, she will speak with them. This may have secondary gain for Jenny, as many of the girls in her class ask to be invited over to hear her speak. When in school, however, she does not talk.

Jenny's father is a successful businessman who travels a great deal, much to Jenny's disappointment. Her mother has had intermittent difficulties with anxiety and panic, and successfully takes an SSRI for this.

The treatment of Jenny involved decreasing secondary gain for not talking (education of her classmates and a preset schedule for play dates), requesting her sister not to speak for her, and family involvement in making expectations clear (especially from both her mother and her father). Paternal attention seemed particularly helpful in reinforcing expectations and helping Jenny get attention from her father in an adaptive manner. Additionally, an SSRI was initiated for treatment of anxiety. The combination of treatments was effective in allowing Jenny to begin to speak in school and in public.

Tic Disorders

· ·

 Tourette Disorder and Other Tic Disorders

Essential Concepts
- Motor tics are repetitive, involuntary movements of discrete muscle groups.
- Phonic (or vocal) tics are involuntary sounds.
- The tics of Tourette disorder are temporarily suppressible and preceded by a premonitory urge.
- The tics associated with Tourette disorder characteristically wax and wane.
- High emotions typically exacerbate tics.

CLINICAL DESCRIPTION

There are four tic disorders described in the Diagnostic and Statistical Manual (DSM-IV-TR): 1) Tourette disorder (also known as Tourette syndrome or TS); 2) chronic motor or vocal tic disorder; 3) transient tic disorder; and 4) tic disorder not otherwise specified. Tourette disorder (which will be referred to as TS) is an inherited neurological disorder with onset in childhood, characterized by the presence of multiple motor tics and at least one phonic (vocal) tic. The tics characteristically wax and wane. TS was once considered a rare and bizarre syndrome, with a psychogenic cause. The eponym for the disorder was bestowed by Jean-Martin Charcot on behalf of his resident, Georges Gilles de la Tourette, a French neurologist who published an account of nine patients with the unusual movement disorder in 1885.

For chronic motor or vocal tic disorder, there are single or multiple motor or vocal tics, but not both. Transient tic disorder is single or multiple motor and/or vocal tics for no more than 12 consecutive months. For all of the tic disorders, the tics must occur many times a day, nearly every day, and there must never be a tic-free period of more than three consecutive months. The disturbance must cause distress and impairment and have an onset before the age of 18.

Epidemiology

Estimates of the disorder have increased over time, with the ascertainment of milder forms of tics. It is estimated that 1–10 per 1,000 children suffer from a diagnosable tic disorder. A large, community-based study suggested that over 19% of school-aged children have had tics of some type, with almost 4% of children in regular education fulfilling the diagnostic criteria for TS. As many as 1 in 100 people may experience some form of tic disorder, which includes transient tics, chronic tics, or TS. Males are affected three to four times more often than females. This number decreases in adulthood, as the tic symptoms frequently resolve in the milder forms of the disorder.

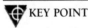 KEY POINT

Coprolalia (the spontaneous utterance of socially objectionable or curse words or phrases) is the most publicized symptom of Tourette disorder, but it is not required for a diagnosis of TS. Fewer than 15% of TS patients exhibit coprolalia.

 TIP

Children with TS describe "premonitory sensory phenomena" or a vague, although sometimes powerful, feeling of needing to tic. Some children liken the feeling to the "need to sneeze" or to "scratch an itch." They are able to suppress the urge for a period of time, but the need to tic seems to build up as irresistible tension. Performing the tic tends to relieve the tension, at least for a time. High levels of either positive or negative emotions tend to exacerbate tics. Concentration in an absorbing activity often leads to a decrease in tics. There are surgeons with TS. They are able to suppress tics for long periods of time for very complex procedures.

Etiology

Genetic studies have proven that the overwhelming majority of cases of TS are inherited. Recent research suggests that a small number of TS cases may be caused by a defect on chromosome 13 of gene SLITRK1. TS is most likely the result of an additive model involving multiple genes in most affected individuals.

The inherited vulnerability to tic disorders may produce varying symptoms in different family members. A person with TS has about a 50% chance of passing the genes to one of his or her children. The genes may express as TS, as a milder tic disorder, or as obsessive-compulsive symptoms with no tics at all. Boys are more likely to demonstrate tics, and females are more likely to demonstrate obsessive-compulsive (OCD) symptoms. Only a minority of the children who inherit the genes will have symptoms severe enough to require medical attention.

While a genetic mechanism is clear, for at least some children with the disorder the exact mechanism has not been established. Research presents considerable evidence that abnormal activity of the brain neurotransmitter, dopamine is involved. Neuroanatomic models implicate abnormalities in the complex cycling cascade of dopaminergic neuronal functions and influences between the brain's cortex and subcortex (especially the striatum and thalamus).

Other factors that have been implicated include perinatal events, such as low birth weight, maternal stress, and obstetric complications. Autoimmune processes may affect tic onset and exacerbation in some cases; the unproven but interesting hypothesis that pediatric autoimmune neuropsychiatric disorders associated with streptococcal infections (PANDAS) play a role in the onset of tic disorders and OCD is a current focus of research.

Assessment

The assessment includes a standard complete psychiatric evaluation. Neurological disorders, such as hyperkinetic movement disorders, including stereotypic behavior, dystonias, choreiform disorders, and myoclonus, may be confused with tics, and should be ruled out (Table 10.1).

Comorbidity and Differential Diagnosis

Individuals with TS are at increased risk of suffering from other psychiatric disorders. The most common comorbidities

TABLE 10.1. Assessment Essentials for Tic Disorders

1. The chief complaint should be obtained from the child and guardian to guide a successful postevaluation discussion and treatment plan formulation.
2. History gathering should include questions that differentiate tics from other movement disorders or stereotypic movements of autism spectrum disorders or stereotyped movement disorder. Ask about "saw tooth" symptom pattern with episodic presentation with abrupt onset and gradual spontaneous reduction associated with group A beta-hemolytic streptococcal infection suggestive of PANDAS.
3. A directed interview will include questions about premonitory urges and ability to temporarily suppress the movements. Additionally, ask questions targeting comorbid conditions, with particular emphasis on symptoms of OCD, ADHD, and learning problems. Testing to rule out learning disorder should be considered if it is suspected.
4. The physical examination should focus on cutaneous abnormalities (suggestive of neurofibromatosis), infectious conditions, and the general neurological exam.
5. Uncomplicated and classical tic disorders do not require other extensive testing. However, for concerns about a movement disorder inconsistent with tics, neuroimaging may be required. Laboratory testing should occur when considering possible metabolic or infectious causes. If PANDAS are implicated, antistreptococcal antibody levels should be drawn.

are OCD and attention deficit hyperactivity disorder (ADHD). Learning disabilities, sleep disorders, disruptive behavior disorders, and mood disorders may also complicate the clinical condition of children and adolescents with TS.

Treatment

TS is a complex and variable disorder in terms of severity and functional disability. Knowledge, understanding, and support are some of the best treatments for tics. The child may be frightened and humiliated by the symptoms. Teachers may not understand the behaviors. Helping educate children and adults alike can go a very long way in terms of destigmatizing the disorder and helping the child avoid the assaults to self-esteem that many children with TS suffer (Table 10.2).

TABLE 10.2. Essentials of Treatment for Tic Disorders

Psychosocial Treatments

Parent and child psychoeducation—education about the disorder for the child and family helps destigmatize and decrease secondary depression, avoidance, and behavioral problems. Additionally, stress reduction and family treatment may be useful to decrease high levels of anxiety or emotion.

Behavioral intervention—habit reversal training (HRT) is a specific and evidence-based behavioral technique used to reduce repetitive behavior by a cooperative and invested child or adolescent. This involves awareness of tics, learning a competitive motor behavior instead of the tic, relaxation techniques, and positive feedback for improvements.

Supportive psychotherapy—this may be helpful for a child who is struggling with issues of self-esteem and other tic- or non-tic–related issues.

Educational/School Related Interventions

Psychoeducational assessment—cognitive and academic assessment is recommended if learning disorders are suspected.

Teacher and class psychoeducation—helping classroom teachers and the other students understand the disorder to minimize teasing or being ostracized may be very helpful in terms of social functioning and self-esteem.

Medication Treatment for Tics

Alpha-2a agonists (first line)
  Clonidine, guanfacine
Neuroleptics
  Atypical (second line)
  Risperidone, ziprasidone
  Typical (third line)
  Pimozide,[a] haloperidol
Nicotine receptor antagonist (neuroleptic augmentation)
  Mecamylamine

[a]Black box warning for potential of prolonged cardiac conduction (QTc).

Medication treatment of tics plus ADHD is complicated because stimulant medication and bupropion may exacerbate tics. If there is significant and impairing ADHD, however, stimulant medications can be used cautiously. Several studies have shown that stimulants do not exacerbate tics any more than placebo does. However, the "start low and go slow" advice remains. Be advised that the Physicians Desk Reference does include an FDA warning that stimulants should not be used in the presence of tic disorders. Atomoxetine and tricyclic antidepressants may be effective if alpha agonists and stimulant medications do not appropriately treat a severe tic disorder with ADHD.

CASE VIGNETTE

Toby is a 6-year-old boy referred by his pediatrician to you after work-up revealed no medical etiology for Toby's recurrent dry cough. His mother was initially concerned and then annoyed with his repetitive cough, which she described "as though he's forcing it to happen or something." This cough seemed unrelated to runny nose or any illness. It had gone on for months at a time—just when his mother thought it was going away, it would re-emerge. Additionally, Toby was hyperactive and inattentive. His teacher noted that he could not sit still in his seat, he blurted out answers, could not wait his turn, and seemed as though "his motor was running on high speed." She also noted that Toby had an eye-blinking habit that the other children had noticed and some began to mimic.

On examination, Toby was an attractive and well-developed 6-year-old boy, who had a knack for precarious acrobatics in the waiting room and in the office. He presented as bright and articulate, but quite hypermotoric. Neurological examination was essentially normal. There were periods of rapid eye blinking and a dry cough. Toby's father displayed subtle sniffing and eye-blinking movements. Family history was positive for a paternal grandmother who was a "control freak" and did not let anyone sit on the white furniture in the living room. Toby's father and paternal uncle had ADHD.

You diagnose a tic disorder (not yet TS, as it has not been a year) and ADHD. You set up the following treatment plan:

1. Education about TS as a disorder, the cause, and the treatments. You stress that many children never need medication for TS, although there are medications if the symptoms are severe. You discuss the possibility of a mild tic disorder in the father, as well. You discuss the fact that TS and ADHD often occur together.
2. Further evaluation, including school-based evaluation (cognitive and academic) to rule out learning disability. You talk to school personnel about the tic disorder and how to talk about the tic disorder with other students.

You discuss with the school social worker the possibility of having a session on medical disorders (such as TS, diabetes, etc.) for the other students so that they may understand Toby better. The school sets a strict policy about teasing and ensures that students who mimic Toby are educated about TS and about the harmful effects of teasing. You send ADHD scales to the teacher. You have the parents fill out an ADHD scale. You consider the need for a Section 504 plan for extra support services for Toby's ADHD and tic disorder.

3. Behavioral structure and support plan at home for ADHD symptoms, including structure, consistency, decreased stimulation, and opportunities for "noncontingent" positive regard and engagement.

4. Pharmacologic intervention with guanfacine or clonidine, which may address hyperkinesis and tics, or atomoxetine for the treatment of ADHD. If severe and functionally impairing ADHD symptoms persist, consider a "start low and go slow" trial of a stimulant medication.

PART E
Elimination Disorders

. . . .

 Elimination Disorders:
Functional Encopresis
and Functional Enuresis

> **Essential Concepts**
> - A biological etiology must be ruled out in all cases of enuresis and encopresis.
> - Nocturnal enuresis may be developmental and tends to run in families.
> - New onset of nocturnal or daytime enuresis or encopresis in a child that has previously been toilet trained needs to be investigated for medical issues as well as trauma or severe psychosocial stress.

CLINICAL DESCRIPTION

Elimination disorders first come to the attention of pediatricians when a child is having difficulty with toilet training. Children are toilet trained at widely different times depending upon development, culture, and techniques utilized to help the child learn. Functional encopresis is fecal soiling in clothes or inappropriate places at least once monthly for at least 3 months in a child that is 4 years old or older, when full bowel control is developmentally expected. Functional enuresis is repeated voiding of urine during the day or at night at least twice weekly for at least 3 months, causing functional impairment and with an age (chronological or mental age) of at least 5 years.

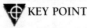 KEY POINT

Some children do not learn to use the toilet within an expected time frame. This is called primary enuresis or encopresis.

Children who are toilet trained but revert back to soiling or urinating during the day or at night after being continent for at least 1 year are said to exhibit secondary enuresis or encopresis. Both sets of disorders require a medical workup to rule out medical causes.

 TIP

Extreme stress or abuse (particularly sexual abuse), as well as a new onset medical condition (such as diabetes), should be suspected and assessed in all cases of secondary enuresis or encopresis.

FUNCTIONAL ENCOPRESIS

Encopresis typically occurs during the day. Many children may deny soiling, even when stool is discovered in their underwear or the odor is obvious. Primary encopresis constitutes about half of the cases and is more common with boys with developmental delay. Children with secondary encopresis experience higher levels of psychosocial adversity and may demonstrate conduct problems.

There are two types of encopresis—that with constipation and overflow incontinence (called retentive encopresis), and that without. Children with retentive encopresis often respond positively to treatment of constipation.

Epidemiology

An estimated 1% of 5-year-olds suffer from encopresis, with boys 2.5 to 6 times more commonly affected than girls. Children with lower cognitive functioning and lower socioeconomic status tend to have higher rates as well.

Etiology

Retentive encopresis often starts with a child who has toilet-related fears, inadequate or punitive toilet training, or constipation which makes defecating painful. This may set into motion a cycle of increased avoidance of using the toilet.

When constipation is more severe, colon motility decreases and, in severe cases, megacolon with decreased sensation may result. Liquid stool leaks around the impaction and the child is unaware and unable to exert control. Stress-induced diarrhea may also cause encopresis. Nonretentive encopresis is the deliberate soiling in inappropriate places. Deliberate soiling suggests that the child is experiencing extreme distress which he/she is unable to communicate directly (e.g., anger, fear of abuse, or severe psychosocial stress) or may be secondary to anal masturbation, sexual abuse, or severe conduct issues. Nonretentive encopresis is more difficult to treat.

Assessment

The assessment includes a standard complete psychiatric evaluation. Additionally, a detailed history of bowel function, nature and pattern of soiling, attempts to train or treat, bathroom habits, and environment is needed. This is a prototype disorder for pediatric–child and adolescent psychiatric collaboration. Physical disorders (Hirschsprung disease or congenital megacolon, irritable bowel or inflammatory bowel disease, thyroid disease, hypercalcemia, lactase deficiency, spina bifida or other neurological disorder, rectal stenosis, anal fissure or anorectal trauma) need to be checked and ruled out.

The psychiatric evaluation includes assessment for associated emotional disorders. Phobic or anxious children may avoid using the toilet (especially in public places), with soiling when they can no longer "hold it." Highly impulsive children with ADHD or other disorders may not stop to go to the bathroom. Oppositional, angry, or abused children may soil willfully. Mentally retarded children may have difficulty with hygiene and have difficulty learning to use the toilet appropriately.

Treatment methods for functional encopresis are provided in Table 11.1.

FUNCTIONAL ENURESIS

Bedwetting is more common than daytime incontinence. Most children achieve daytime bladder control 1 to 2 years prior to nighttime control. It is unusual for a child to display daytime enuresis without nocturnal enuresis. Children with encopresis often also display enuresis. The constipation may lead to vesico-ureteric reflux and chronic urinary tract infections as well.

TABLE 11.1. Treatment of Functional Encopresis

	Retentive Type	*Nonretentive Type*
Medical	Laxatives and bowel cleanout Stool softeners to prevent constipation Cisapride a possible treatment	No specific medical intervention
Education	Educate about bowel function Educate about bowel hygiene	
Psychosocial	Relaxation training Regular toileting routine Behavioral treatment Biofeedback Psychotherapy for associated disorders	Behavioral shaping Regular toileting routine Parent-management training Assessment and treatment if abuse or high environmental stress Individual and family therapy

There are three types of enuresis: nocturnal only, diurnal only, and both nocturnal and diurnal. Primary enuresis (85%) is more common than secondary (15%) enuresis.

Epidemiology

An estimated 5 to 10% of 5-year-olds and around 3 to 5% of 10-year-olds suffer from enuresis. This rate decreases to 1% by adolescence and adulthood. Boys display more primary enuresis than girls. For both boys and girls, there is a spontaneous decline of 5 to 10% of cases per year. Secondary enuresis has similar incidence in boys and girls.

Etiology

There seems to be a strong genetic factor for primary enuresis. Approximately 70% of children with enuresis (especially boys) have a first-degree relative with functional enuresis.

It may be "maturational," as children with primary enuresis tend to have small-volume voiding, low mean bone age, delayed sexual maturation, and short stature. The relationship between emotional upset and enuresis is not clear. Children with anxiety disorders may avoid bathrooms, with resulting incontinence. Children with ADHD tend to have higher rates of enuresis. The relationship between sleep architecture and nocturnal enuresis is unclear, but under investigation.

Assessment

Initial medical evaluation is required to rule out medical causes (urinary tract infection, urethritis, diabetes mellitus and insipidus, sickle cell trait, seizure disorder, neurogenic bladder, genitourinary abnormality, some medications). Family history should concentrate on other family members with a history of enuresis, as well as on family history of diabetes or renal disease.

The psychiatric evaluation should concentrate on the assessment of associated psychiatric symptoms (especially anxiety and ADHD), recent psychosocial stressors or trauma, and family concern about management of the symptoms. Early psychoeducation should stress low emotionality toward the child when he wets and helping the child learn to care

TABLE 11.2. Treatment of Functional Enuresis

	Nocturnal	Diurnal
Medical	Bladder training	Bladder training
	Bell and pad	TCA
	Desmopressin	
	Tricyclic antidepressant	
Educational	Hygiene and cleanliness training	Hygiene and cleanliness training
	Fluid restriction at night	
	Waking the child to void in the night	
Psychosocial	Monitoring and reward for staying dry	Behavioral program
	Avoid punishment or ridicule	Regular toileting times
	Psychotherapy for associated disorders	Psychotherapy for associated disorders

for himself. Additionally, addressing issues of distress, embarrassment, and affront to self-esteem is required.

The medications used to treat nocturnal enuresis include tricyclic antidepressants (usually imipramine) and desmopressin (DDAVP), which is an analog to antidiuretic hormone and decreases urine output. The bell and pad is a devise that sounds an alarm when it becomes damp. When a child urinates in his sleep, the alarm sounds and wakes up the child and family. Through a classical conditioning paradigm, the child then begins to wake up spontaneously before voiding.

Treatment methods for functional enuresis are provided in Table 11.2.

PART F
Feeding and Eating Disorders
of Infancy or Early Childhood
· ·

12

Feeding and Eating
Disorders of Infancy or
Early Childhood: Pica,
Rumination Disorder,
Feeding Disorder of Infancy
or Early Childhood

Essential Concepts
- Pica, the eating of non-nutritive substances, may be normative in very young children, but increases the risk of lead poisoning.
- Rumination disorder of infancy is a rare, but potentially fatal eating disorder in the first year of life.
- Feeding disorder of infancy or early childhood is what had historically been called psychosocial dwarfism or failure to thrive.
- All feeding and eating disorders require a full medical workup for etiology.

CLINICAL DESCRIPTION

Feeding and eating disorders of infancy or early childhood are typically diagnosed and treated by primary care physicians. There are few maladies that are more upsetting than an infant who is not thriving. Collaboration between the primary care physician, the child's caretakers, and mental health professionals is essential to optimize prognosis. In severe cases, infants die from malnutrition or the secondary consequences of rumination.

Infants who have had multiple caregivers, neglect or abuse, and suboptimal care and bonding are at higher risk of eating disorders. However, in some cases, the cause is never elucidated.

 KEY POINT

The eating disorders typically come to the attention of child and adolescent psychiatrists when they are quite severe and the psychosocial and interactional difficulties are obvious. These disorders require multidisciplinary and very close collaboration between mental health professionals, pediatric care specialists, and frequently protective services, to ensure the safety of the child and optimal outcomes of treatment.

PICA

Pica is the eating of non-nutritive substances on a persistent basis for at least 1 month. This behavior must not be developmentally appropriate and not part of a culturally sanctioned practice.

Pica is most commonly seen in very young children. It may be culturally sanctioned in some cultures for pregnant women to eat bricks or clay. For children, the rates are increased with mental retardation and pervasive developmental disorders. For individuals with severe mental retardation, the rate of pica may be as high as 15%. Vitamin deficiencies have been postulated as a cause, and a minority of cases may have a mineral deficiency (e.g., zinc). Children with pica also eat nutritive foods, so they do not typically suffer from malnutrition. The most serious complications of pica are lead poisoning from eating paint chips, mechanical bowel obstruction from eating hair or other nondigestibles, and toxoplasmosis or other parasites from eating feces or dirt. Poverty, neglect, and developmental delay increase the risk of pica.

 KEY POINT

Before the age of 24 months, mouthing and eating of non-nutritive substances is fairly common and does not imply pica. However, it is essential to ensure that caretakers are supervising carefully, as infants may choke or get lead poisoning from their ingestions.

TABLE 12.1. Comparison of Rumination Disorder and Feeding Disorder of Infancy

	Rumination Disorder	Feeding Disorder of Infancy or Early Childhood
Definition	After a period of normal eating, child repeatedly regurgitates and rechews, not due to GI problem	Persistent failure to eat adequately, resulting in weight loss or failure to gain, not due to GI problem; before age 6
Epidemiology	Rare	3% of children have failure to thrive; males = females
Etiology	Unknown—increased risk with mother with eating disorder, gastroesophageal reflux, MR, developmental delay, medical illness	Child temperament, developmental impairments that make the infant less responsive; environmental factors of parental psychopathology and child abuse or neglect
Differential diagnosis	Gastrointestinal disorders	Gastrointestinal, endocrinological, or neurological conditions
Treatment	Parent training in behavioral techniques—positive attention and interaction, ignoring ruminative behavior; may require hospitalization and alternative feeding environment; reassurance, education, and support of parents	Support for attachment and bonding, parent–child interactional therapy, parent training in behavioral techniques; may require hospitalization for treatment of malnutrition

RUMINATION DISORDER AND FEEDING DISORDER OF INFANCY OR EARLY CHILDHOOD

These eating disorders are complex and multidetermined disorders. In general, parent-child interactional deficits are assumed, although this may not always be evident. We believe that the disorders may be multidetermined—typically with a developmental or temperamental issue of the child and a poor fit with the nurturing environment (Table 12.1).

Fortunately, ruminative disorder is rare, but it can be fatal. Feeding disorder of infancy or early childhood is variable in its severity—from mild and temporary, to severe and potentially fatal. The majority of children have improved growth, although they may remain shorter and weigh less through adolescence than their peers.

 TIP

Take a deep breath before starting one of these cases. It is quite emotionally intense, the potential for treatment splitting and disagreement is high, and the negative feelings toward parents of these infants who are literally wasting away can be counterproductive. Be sure that you have a multidisciplinary team and talk about and work out the emotional and "splitting" issues, in addition to following the weight of the child.

III

**GENERAL
PSYCHIATRIC
DISORDERS THAT
MAY BEGIN IN
CHILDHOOD OR
ADOLESCENCE**

Depressive Disorders: Major Depression, Dysthymia, Depression NOS

Essential Concepts
Screening Questions
- Have you felt down or depressed?
- Have your friends noticed a change in you?
- Have you lost interest in things you used to like to do?
- Have you been feeling that life will never get better?

Mnemonic: SIG: E-CAPS

Our generation has had no Great War, no Great Depression. Our war is spiritual. Our depression is our lives.

—Chuck Palahniuk

CLINICAL DESCRIPTION

Rates of depression have increased over the past five decades, with younger age of onset. Many adolescents suffer from brief periods of depression when they are faced with an upsetting event or disappointment (breakup with girlfriend or boyfriend, for example). With increased rates of depressive disorders has come an increased rate of suicide attempts. However, after a marked increase, the rates of completed suicides for youth have declined since 1990, possibly due to improved detection and intervention of depression. Substance use, concomitant conduct problems, and impulsivity increase risk.

Major depressive disorder (MDD) and dysthymic disorder (DD) in children and adolescents are diagnosed in the same manner as those of adults. However, children and adolescents may present differently. Irritability, the new onset of opposition-ality and angry outbursts, and failure to make expected weight gain may be indicative of depression in children and adolescents. A rather precipitous drop in grades may be a clue to diminished interest and motivation and difficulty concentrating. Depressed mood and/or loss of interest or pleasure are key characteristics of MDD. Neurovegetative symptoms are those that suggest physical manifestations of the depression. Symptoms must be present for at least 2 weeks and must be functionally impairing to make a diagnosis of major depression.

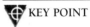 KEY POINT

One of the most difficult parts of psychiatry is asking the uncomfortable questions. Asking about suicide is one of those questions. However, put it into your repertoire of questions that you ask all children and adolescents. You may save a life.

MAJOR DEPRESSIVE EPISODE (MDD)

Mnemonic: SIG E CAPS

When checking for neurovegetative symptoms of depression, think of the mnemonic devised by Dr. Carey Gross at MGH which refers to what one might write on a prescription sheet for a depressed patient: **SIG**: **E**nergy **CAPS**ules

Sleep disorder (either increased or decreased)*
Interest deficit (anhedonia)
Guilt (worthlessness,* hopelessness,* regret)
Energy deficit*
Concentration deficit*
Appetite disorder (either decreased or increased)*
Psychomotor retardation or agitation
Suicidality

*For dysthymia, two of the six starred symptoms must be present for a 1-year duration.

CLINICAL VIGNETTE

A 15-year-old adolescent girl presented for her first office visit because her parents are concerned that she is depressed. You ask about sad mood and find out that she has been crying every day since she broke up with her boyfriend over 2 weeks ago. She has not wanted to get out of bed, and her friends have complained that she doesn't want to go out with them anymore. She has typically been an A–B student and failed her first math test last week. You ask if she has felt as though life was no longer worth living, and she replies, "Sure, but it doesn't do any good. I took 10 Tylenols last week and I'm still here." You assess for acute suicidality and ask her mother to join the session. The girl tells her mother, who responds with appropriate concern. You determine the patient is safe to go home, but her mother will secure all medications. You send her to get blood drawn for liver function tests due to potential hepatoxicity of acetaminophen, and add thyroid and basic screening labs to the panel. You call her pediatrician to inform her of the patient's depression and overdose. You set up the patient for a partial hospital program the next day.

Epidemiology

The prevalence of MDD is approximately 2% in preadolescent children, with a roughly equal prevalence of boys and girls. In adolescents, the prevalence is approximately 6%, with a female-to-male ratio of 2:1, similar to the adult population. Population-based studies estimate lifetime prevalence rates of MDD by age 19 to be 28% (35% in young women and 19% in young men). The average duration of an untreated major depressive episode in a child or adolescent is 7 to 9 months. Unfortunately, 50% of youth relapse. About 10% will have a chronic course. Prevalence rates for DD are similar to MDD: 0.6 to 1.7% in children and 1.6 to 8.0% in adolescents.

It is increasingly clear that depression is often a chronic, recurrent disorder likely to continue into adulthood. Comorbid psychiatric disorders (especially conduct disorder), exposure to negative life events, family history of MDD, and conflict within the youth's family all lead to a worse prognosis. Additionally, 20 to 40% of those with childhood-onset MDD with psychotic features, family history of bipolar disorder, or a hypomanic episode as a result of antidepressant medications will develop bipolar disorder.

CLINICAL VIGNETTE

A resident was interviewing a 17-year-old twelfth-grade adolescent and asked, "How have you been sleeping?" The youth answered, "Terribly. I never get to sleep until 1:00 or 2:00 and then I can't get out of bed in the morning." The resident considered this statement sufficient to meet the criteria for the insomnia of depression, until the girl mentioned that she has been a "night owl" since ninth grade, preferring to stay up at night Instant-Messaging with friends. It turned out that she had a sleep cycle disorder (common in adolescents).

Etiology

The etiology of depression is not completely understood. We know that the following factors play a role: genetic heritability, dysregulation of central serotonergic or noradrenergic systems, hypothalamic-pituitary-adrenal (HPA) axis dysfunction, and the influence of pubertal sex hormones. Personality factors such as a negative cognitive style have been implicated. Individuals with negative cognitive styles tend to see the "glass half empty" in all situations and see little positive in their lives. The stress-diathesis model suggests that a negative cognitive style combined with negative life events and environmental adversity is contributory to MDD.

Assessment

When assessing the child or adolescent who may be depressed, it is important to perform a comprehensive psychiatric evaluation that considers all possible psychiatric disorders, as symptoms of depression overlap with other disorders (Table 13.1). One should also be alert to the possibility of mania, as juvenile bipolar disorder frequently presents with a mixed state of depressive and manic symptoms.

 TIP

Contracting for safety is a good way to engage children and adolescents around their responsibility for safety. However, don't put too much faith in them. There is no evidence that "safety contracts" protect against suicide. Listen to the patient's behavior as much as the words.

TABLE 13.1. Assessment Essentials for Depression

1. The clinical interview remains the most accurate method for assessing the presence of depression.
2. Interview the child or adolescent separately to obtain accurate information about depressive symptoms.
3. Rating scales may be used as adjunctive measures to elicit more information about symptoms (such as the Beck Depression Inventory [DBI] or the Childhood Depression Inventory [CDI]).
4. Assessment of suicidality is an essential component of the assessment of depression.
5. Both the parents and the youth should be asked about the presence of suicide risk factors, including the availability of guns, large quantities of medications, or other potential methods of suicide.
6. Comorbid conditions such as anxiety disorders, substance abuse, and disruptive behavior disorders should be evaluated.
7. Physical examination, review of systems, and laboratory testing should be done to rule out medical causes (e.g., anemia, infectious illness, hypothyroidism, effects of illicit substances or medications).

KEY POINT

Successful intervention for suicidal behavior in youths targets three domains: 1) treatment of current psychopathology; 2) remediation of social, problem-solving, and affective regulation deficits; and 3) family psychoeducation and intervention.

Treatment

Treatment is multimodal and requires a thoughtful, stepwise intensive treatment of the child and adolescent. Table 13.2 gives the essentials of treatment, elaborating on the types of psychosocial and medication treatment options available. Figure 13.1 suggests an algorithm for acute treatment of major depression.

There has been much recent controversy about the use of SSRIs and other antidepressants in children and adolescents. The data suggest that antidepressants pose a 4% risk, versus a 2% risk in placebo, of suicidal thinking or behavior. This prompted the FDA to issue a "black box" warning for

TABLE 13.2. Essentials of Multimodal Treatment of Depression

Ensuring Safety

Parent and child psychoeducation—about depression as a disease, treatments, and what the patient and family can do to decrease depression. Education around safety—need to secure medications. Always ask about guns and be sure there are none or they are locked.

Hospitalization—If the youth is suicidal or engaging in self-destructive behaviors, hospitalization needs to be considered.

Partial hospital and therapeutic after-school programs—If the risk is not imminent, but safety and severity of depression is of concern, Partial Hospital and Therapeutic After-School Programs may be considered.

Environmental stress—Identify and minimize stressors. Refer parents with their own depression or other mental health issues for treatment as well.

Collaboration with primary care physician—Monitor and collaborate in ensuring overall health (mental and physical) of the child is being treated.

School psychoeducation—with consent, close collaboration between outside treaters and school personnel is advised. School counseling and outpatient therapy should be coordinated with a unified treatment approach.

Psychosocial Treatments

Cognitive-behavioral treatment (CBT)—strongest evidence of effectiveness. Identifies patient's cognitive distortions and promotes more realistic and positive cognitions.

Interpersonal therapy (ITP)—focuses on problematic styles of interaction that may be a symptom of or a contributor to depression.

Supportive psychotherapy—helps the child reconnect with prior coping skills and restore a sense of hopefulness.

Behavior therapy—focuses on changing behaviors that may fuel depression. A focus on lifestyle (exercise, getting out, etc.) may be particularly helpful.

Family therapy—engaging families and working directly with family relationship and communication difficulties are critical to treating depressed youth.

Psychodynamic psychotherapy—talking (or play therapy for younger children). Most helpful for chronic dysthymia and highly motivated patients (and their families) who are capable of insight.

(Continued)

TABLE 13.2. Essentials of Multimodal Treatment of Depression (*continued*)

Group therapy—many children and adolescents prefer a group experience. Can be helpful for support, psychoeducation. Beware of discussions about self-destructive behavior and "copycat" behaviors.

Medication Treatment for Depression

Selective serotonin reuptake Inhibitors (SSRIs)

Fluoxetine (Prozac)	8 and older (for MDD, OCD)
Sertraline (Zoloft)	6 and older (for OCD)
Fluvoxamine (Luvox)	8 and older (for OCD)
Citalopram (Celexa)	18 and older
Escitalopram (Lexapro)	18 and older
Paroxetine (Paxil)	18 and older
Other antidepressants	
Clomipramine (Anafranil)	8 and older (for OCD)
Bupropion (Wellbutrin)	18 and
Mirtazepine (Remeron)	18 and older
Nefazadone (Serzone)	18 and older
Trazodone (Desyrel)	18 and older
Venlafaxine (Effexor)	18 and older

All antidepressants have a "black box" warning for potential increases in suicidality. Only fluoxetine is FDA approved for use in children for major depression.

suicidality for all of the antidepressants. Notably, there were no completed suicides in the study samples. Fluoxetine, the best studied of the medications, is the only one to show a significant advantage over placebo in terms of efficacy for major depression in children and adolescents (although citalopram has some positive studies, as well).

Although we do not entirely understand the finding of increased "suicidality," activation is a noted side effect of the selective serotonin reuptake inhibitors (SSRIs), and may result in more acting-out behavior. The increased energy that is noted as depression lifts, but before the patient experiences significant emotional relief, may also increase the potential of self-harm behavior. The risk of "switching" of children who are predisposed, from depression to mania, must always be considered.

In an effort to improve safety and ensure that patients with major depression receive effective treatment, the following is recommended for monitoring:

**Acute Treatment of MDD
Mild-Moderate Episode**
(few if any symptoms in excess to make diagnosis, mild to
moderate functional impairment)

---

1. Start with psychoeducation and psychotherapy (for 4–6 weeks).
2. If only partial or no response, continue psychoeducation, psychotherapy, and start SSRI (continue for 6–12 weeks).
3. If no response after 6–12 weeks, switch to another SSRI (continue for 6–12 weeks).
4. If no response after 6–12 weeks of second SSRI, recheck diagnosis/comorbidities (especially ADHD and anxiety), adherence/compliance, medical illnesses, family functioning, negative life events, parent/sibling illness. Consider referral to specialist. May switch to a second-line antidepressant (buproprion, venlafaxine, nefazodone, mirtazapine).
5. Continue medication for 6–12 months after a response, then, if no relapse, progressively discontinue treatment.
6. If a second uncomplicated episode, then continue medication for 1–3 years.

**Acute Treatment of MDD
Severe Episode**
(several symptoms in excess of those to make diagnosis and
symptoms markedly interfere with functioning, suicidality,
psychotic features, bipolar, and/or recurrent)

---

1. Start with psychoeducation, psychotherapy, and an SSRI (for 4–6 weeks). If suicidality is present, consider safety issues and level of care.
2. If no response after 6–12 weeks, switch to another SSRI (continue for 6–12 weeks).
3. If no response after 6–12 weeks, consider referral to specialist or switch to a second-line antidepressant (buproprion, venlafaxine, nefazodone, mirtazapine).
4. Continue medication for 1–3 years.
5. If two or more complicated depressive episodes, three or more uncomplicated episodes, or chronic depression, then continue medication for 3 years to lifelong.

FIG. 13.1. Suggested algorithm for acute treatment of major depression. (Reprinted with permission from Cheng K, Myers KM. *Child and Adolescent Psychiatry: The Essentials.* Philadelphia, PA, Lippincott Williams & Wilkins, 2005.)

1. Discuss risks (including suicidal and self-destructive behavior) with parents, guardians, and patients. Advise parents what symptoms (increased agitation, thoughts of suicide, or anxiety and restlessness) to look for and to call right away if these new symptoms occur.
2. Set up weekly monitoring visits for the first month, then twice monthly for a month, and at least monthly thereafter.

The most important aspect of treating depressed children and youth is engaging them and their families actively in treatment, and providing the intensive, closely supervised treatment necessary to decrease suffering and improve prognosis.

Juvenile Onset Bipolar Disorder

Essential Concepts
Screening Questions
- Have you had periods of time when you feel so happy and energetic that you feel "on top of the world" or as if you could do anything?
- Have you had periods of time when your friends said you are talking too much or too fast?
- Has there been a period when you were so hyper and irritable that you got into lots of arguments with people?

Mnemonic: DIGFAST

Initially thought to be only a disorder of adolescence or adulthood, bipolar disorder (BD) is now increasingly being recognized and diagnosed in prepubertal children. Considerable ambiguity remains about the actual prevalence of BD in children. Lifetime prevalence of BD is estimated at 1%. A point prevalence of mania in 14- to 16-year-olds of 0.6% was identified by Carlson and Kashani. The comorbidity with ADHD has also not been established, although data suggest it may be common (around 30%). Some symptoms (high levels of activity, talkativeness, appears as if powered by a motor) may be similar, and it is important to differentiate a mood component in the differential diagnosis. Other frequent comorbidities are conduct disorder, substance abuse disorders, anxiety disorders, trauma-induced disorders, and borderline personality disorder traits. Schizophrenia may be confused with bipolar disorder. Although BD in adults tends to be gender neutral, it is estimated that prepubertal BD is almost four times more frequently diagnosed in boys. Compared with adults, children and adolescents with BD may have a more prolonged early course and be less responsive to treatment.

CLINICAL DESCRIPTION

Bipolar I disorder requires the existence of a manic or mixed episode. A manic episode is defined in the DSM-IV-TR as a distinct period of "abnormally and persistently elevated, expansive, or irritable mood." A mixed episode is characterized by "rapidly alternating mood with symptoms of a manic episode and a major depressive episode." Children with manic episodes may not present with the same discrete periods seen in adults. Early onset bipolar disorder has been described as highly variable, often with a rapid-cycling, chronic, nonepisodic presentation. Additionally, irritability and unpredictable, labile mood and psychotic features may be more common in young people presenting with the disease.

Bipolar II disorder includes major depressive episodes alternating with hypomanic episodes. Hypomania may present as elevated, expansive, or irritable mood, which is less severe and less functionally impairing than a manic episode.

Cyclothymic disorder is a chronic and fluctuating mood disorder, with hypomanic and depressive symptoms that are less functionally impairing that BD and that have been persistent for a year.

 KEY POINT

Early onset BD often begins with an episode of depression, not mania. It is estimated that 20 to 40% of youth will "switch" to BD within 5 years of depression. Features associated with "switching" include early onset depression, psychomotor retardation, psychosis, mood lability, seasonal pattern, family history of BD or mood disorders, and antidepressant-induced hypomania.

Diagnosis of Manic Episode

A mnemonic that is helpful in recalling the essential features of mania is **DIGFAST**. The term may refer to the speed with which a manic patient would dig a hole if put to the task, as they may appear as if "driven by a motor." At least three symptoms are required (four if mood is only irritable):

Distractibility
Indiscretion (excessive involvement in pleasurable activities that are likely to have adverse consequences)
Grandiosity or inflated self-esteem
Flight of ideas or racing thoughts
Activity increase (increase in goal-directed activity or psychomotor agitation)
Sleep deficit
Talkativeness or pressured speech

A manic episode must last at least a week or be severe enough to require hospitalization.

KEY POINT

The usual adult psychiatric interview to discuss manic and depressive episodes generally does not work with children. The onset of the disorder may be more insidious; the presentation may be "atypical" with psychotic symptoms, suicidal attempts, and serious acting-out behavior that may mask the mood disorder. It is essential to get information from a variety of sources to clarify timelines, specific mood symptoms, sleep patterns, energy level, and course of illness to more clearly clarify the diagnosis.

TIP

Mood lability (rapid mood swings) and rage outbursts in children and adolescents may have many etiologies, including bipolar disorder. The marked increase in the number of prepubertal children being diagnosed with BD is suspect, as it is higher than that expected by epidemiological studies in adults. I have the "Five Stars in Alignment" theory of the increase in diagnosis. Here are the five stars which I feel have "aligned" to substantially increase the number of prepubertal children being diagnosed with bipolar disorder:

1. Children have BD which has gone unrecognized, and we are now beginning to appropriately diagnose these patients;
2. There is a great deal written about the labile child being the bipolar child. Parents find this reassuring, in that there is an actual diagnosis and treatment for the disorder that they have been struggling with;
3. Children like the disorder because it helps deflect punishment of "bad" behavior to that of "ill" behavior ("it's just another manic episode");
4. Psychiatrists like it because it gives a sense of efficacy in treatment. Also, the same medications may be used to treat mood lability and aggression as those for BD;
5. There is insurance parity for bipolar disorder, and payment may be secured for this diagnosis and not for a more nebulous diagnosis associated with aggressive outbursts and labile mood (such as conduct disorder or many others).

CLINICAL VIGNETTE

A 12-year-old boy presented due to a new onset of increased irritability over the past 2 months. He has been talking back to his parents, and when they say, "No" to a request, he flies into a rage. They bring him to your office for an evaluation after he punched and kicked holes in the wall during one of his rages. His family noted an increase in stress in the family—his grandmother, with whom he had been close, died 2 months ago. Additionally, he had an argument with his best friend, and they have not been speaking. He has seemed moody and "on edge" and has not been sleeping well. He was suspended from school last week for disrespectful behavior. You learn that there is a strong family history for mood disorder (his mother is depressed, her brother is bipolar, and his paternal grandfather is an alcoholic and possibly bipolar; his father drinks a great deal). The boy has been taking methylphenidate since age 8 for ADHD with generally good results, although he has always been oppositional and impulsive. You are considering a diagnosis of bipolar disorder. What else do you want to explore? Rule out any medical conditions (e.g., thyroid) or beginning experimentation with substances. His father drinks, his mother is depressed, and his grandmother recently died—is this an atypical grief reaction/major depression, or an adjustment disorder related to domestic violence or other noted stresses? He has ADHD and oppositionality—is this a secondary conduct disorder? School issues—social and academic—need to be explored.

Etiology

Etiology is multifactorial. There is genetic loading for all mood disorders in family members of BD children, some specificity-increased loading of BD, and family loading that is higher for childhood onset than for adolescent onset BD. Earlier onset of BD in adults increases the risk of BD in offspring during childhood or adolescence. Earlier onset disease often has a more chronic and debilitating course (Table 14.1).

A link has been reported between bipolar adults and the serotonin transporter gene. The long (l) allele has been associated with the prophylactic antidepressant response to lithium. The short (s) allele has been identified as a risk factor for suicidal behavior (common in BD) and for pharmacologically

TABLE 14.1. Essentials of Assessment for Early Onset Bipolar Disorder

- Physical examination, review of systems, and laboratory testing to rule out suspected medical etiologies, including neurological, systemic, and substance-induced disorders.
- Interview of parents regarding child's symptoms—timeline, character, and severity. Ask about child risk-taking behaviors (substance use, legal issues, sexual acting out, suicidal/homicidal threats or behavior). Get family genetic history.
- Interview of child/youth—questions, observation, and description of their inner state. Assess thought process, psychotic symptoms, depressive symptoms, anxiety symptoms. Always ask about suicidality/homicidality and risk-taking behavior (substance use, legal issues, sexual acting out). Always ask about a history of trauma.
- School performance and interpersonal relationships should be assessed to determine the youth's functional impairment and educational needs.
- Rating scales may be helpful (e.g., General Behavior Inventory [GBI] and the parent version [GBI-P]; or the Young Mania Rating Scale [Y-MRS] and the parent version [YMRS-P]).

induced mania. There are mixed findings in MRI scans of children and adults with regard to brain structure changes.

The environment potentiates a genetic vulnerability. Environmental and psychological factors, particularly acute and chronic stress, have been implicated in the precipitation of the episodes as well as in prognosis.

KEY POINT

Much is said about the risk of suicide for depressed individuals. However, bipolar disorder is an even higher risk factor. An individual in the throes of grandiosity and feeling good may seem to be at low risk, but high levels of irritability and impulsivity, and poor ability to consider consequences increase risk of completed suicide. Ensuring safety is always the first consideration.

Treatment

Treatment of bipolar disorder includes stabilization of acute symptoms, as well as longer-term stabilization and maintenance.

TABLE 14.2. Essentials of Treatment of Bipolar Disorder

1. Level of care considerations—safety issues are primary.
   Hospitalization for acute safety issues. Partial hospitalization, intensive outpatient treatment, intensive in-home services as needed for stabilization and safety.
2. Medication treatment
   Mood stabilizer—consider family history of response. Lithium and divalproex are the fist-line treatment for episodes of euphoric mania. (Divalproex may be more effective for mixed or rapid cycling. For females, possible risk of polycystic ovary and not to be used if pregnant.)
   Antipsychotic medication can be used during acute mania with or without psychotic symptoms to stabilize mood, ensure safety, and provide sleep. Chronic use may be needed. (Monitor for "hypermetabolic syndrome" with weight gain, increased lipids, and possible risk of diabetes.)
3. Psychosocial treatment
   Psychoeducation about BD, its risks, treatment, prognosis, and complications associated with medication noncompliance.
   Family therapy to stabilize environment and improve prognosis.
   Individual therapy for support. CBT, anger management, or insight-oriented work may be helpful. Ongoing safety assessment.
   Educational—collaboration with school regarding behavioral management, special educational needs, and appropriate individualized educational plan.

Table 14.2 presents essential issues to consider in treatment of early onset bipolar disorder.

Treating comorbid psychiatric disorders must be done carefully. Stimulants may be used to treat comorbid ADHD once the patient has been stabilized on a mood stabilizer. In general, antidepressants should be avoided; but if the youth becomes depressed and is not responsive to other pharmacotherapy, cautious use of antidepressants may be necessary. Carefully monitor for manic "activation" or "switch," as well as suicidality.

Prognosis

Early onset bipolar disorders have a greater chronicity than do adult onset bipolar disorders and are less responsive to treatment. Up to one-third of children with major depression may later be diagnosed with bipolar disorder. Risk factors for poor outcome have been reported to be long episode duration and high prevalence of mixed mania, psychosis, and rapid cycling.

15 Anxiety Disorders: Generalized Anxiety, Phobias, and Obsessive-Compulsive Disorder

---

Essential Concepts
Screening Questions
- Are there things that you are afraid of?
- Do you often feel nervous? Are there particular things that bring this on?
- Do you have thoughts that you can't get out of your head, even though they really bother you? What are they?
- Are there things that you feel that you must do to help you feel less anxious—like washing your hands, checking on something, or counting things?
- Do others consider you a perfectionist?

Do not anticipate trouble, or worry about what may never happen. Keep in the sunlight.

—Benjamin Franklin

CLINICAL DESCRIPTION

Most children experience various fears throughout their childhood, and some of these fears are specific to developmental stage. In contrast to fear, anxiety is defined as an anticipatory response to perceived threat, either internal or external. Both fear and anxiety are characterized by distressing "fight or flight" reactions and a plethora of other physiological responses that may affect multiple systems, such as cardiac, pulmonary, gastrointestinal, and neurological. Anxiety is further characterized by cognitive symptoms, such as feelings of losing control or losing one's mind, unwelcome or intrusive thoughts, inattention, insomnia, and even perceptual disturbances, such as depersonalization or vague visual images. Children who are anxious tend to be frequent doctor visitors, presenting with a variety of vague aches, pains, and physical symptoms that may frustrate health care providers. Separation anxiety disorder and selective mutism, two anxiety disorders that begin in childhood, have been discussed in Chapters 8 and 9. The present chapter will discuss the anxiety disorders of generalized anxiety, phobias, and obsessive-compulsive disorder.

Generalized Anxiety Disorder

Children with generalized anxiety disorder (GAD) worry excessively about upcoming events and occurrences. This worry has continued mostly unabated for at least 6 months. They worry unduly about their academic performance or sporting activities, about being on time, or even about natural disasters such as earthquakes. The worry persists even when the child is not being judged and has always performed well in the past. Because of their anxiety, children may be overly conforming, perfectionistic, and unsure of themselves. They tend to seek approval and need constant reassurance about their performance and social acceptability. The child may appear restless, tense, irritable, or fatigued. Somatic complaints are common.

Phobic Disorders

Phobic disorders are heterogeneous, consisting of specific phobias, which involve a single feared object or situation, or social phobia, a more serious and impairing condition. Phobic disorders need to be differentiated from the normal episodes of fear often seen in childhood. The difference between having a phobic disorder or an age-appropriate episode of fearfulness is based on developmental considerations, the length and intensity of fearful affect, and the severity of accompanying impairment of everyday functioning.

Fear and avoidance occur in response to a specific object or situation in specific phobias. The anxiety is intense and immediate. Animals, natural disasters, blood or injury or enclosed places are common examples of fears that are common in specific phobias. However, when the feared object or situation is not present, the child functions normally.

Social phobia is more common in adults than in children, but it can be quite debilitating.

Children suffering from social phobia have a persistent fear of being embarrassed in social situations, during a performance, or if they have to speak in class or in public, get into a conversation with others, or eat, drink, or write in public. Feelings of anxiety in these situations produce physical reactions such as palpitations, tremors, sweating, diarrhea, blushing, and muscle tension. Social phobia can lead to school refusal with subsequent school failure and even truancy charges. Socially phobic youth frequently avoid all meaningful social relationships. These children do not have a primary social disability (as one might see with an autism spectrum disorder). However, severe avoidance of social situations may seriously impede normal social development.

 TIP

Consider the child's developmental stage prior to making a diagnosis of phobia. Developmentally normative fears include toddlers being terrified by being separated from their parents, and preschool and kindergarten children being frightened by the dark or "monsters" under the bed; fear of dogs and getting hurt is common. School-age children may be scared of using public bathrooms, and teenagers are often afraid of undressing for gym class or giving a speech in class. Age-appropriate fearfulness that does not derail development is not considered a disorder.

Obsessive-Compulsive Disorder

Obsessive-compulsive disorder (OCD) is characterized by recurrent, time-consuming obsessions or compulsive behaviors that cause distress and/or impairment. The obsessions may be repetitive intrusive images, thoughts, or impulses. Often the compulsive behaviors, such as hand-washing or cleaning rituals, are an attempt to displace the obsessive thoughts. There is a strong familial component to OCD, and there is evidence from twin studies of both genetic susceptibility and environmental influences. Tic disorders and OCD may have similar genetic origins, as they tend to co-occur in families. There is evidence that about 10% of the individuals with OCD may have the symptoms precipitated by pediatric autoimmune neuropsychiatric disorders associated with streptococcal infections (PANDAS). Although evidence remains equivocal, antineuronal antibodies formed against the group A beta-hemolytic streptococcal cell wall antigens may cross-react with caudate neural tissue. This should be considered for children whose symptoms correlate with recurrent strep infections. About half of all adults seeking treatment for OCD report that it began in childhood or adolescence.

Epidemiology

As a group, anxiety disorders affect up to 20% of youth up to age 18 years. Clinically, anxiety disorders are diagnosed equally in men and women, but in epidemiologic samples they are more frequently found in women. Generalized anxiety disorder is thought to affect 3 to 6% of youth. Specific phobias affect about 3% of children. Girls tend to suffer from phobias more commonly than boys, but for both genders the disorder wanes with age. Social phobia has been estimated to affect 1% of children and adolescents at any point in time. Lifetime prevalence may be as high as 13%.

Etiology and Risk Factors

Many investigators postulate that children are born with biologically or constitutionally predetermined temperaments, some of which are a liability for the development of anxiety disorders. Familial factors, both genetic and environmental, contribute to anxiety disorders. General anxiety disorder and major depression seem to have the same genetic risk factors. On the basis of new neuroimaging studies, it is hypothesized than anticipatory anxiety is associated with the cingulated portion of the limbic system, phobic avoidance is associated with the prefrontal cortex, and panic is associated with the brainstem. Serotonin receptor site dysregulation is also posited. The biological vulnerabilities are then variably affected by environmental factors to form clinically significant anxiety symptoms. The environmental factors may be diverse, including neurobiological insults, exposure to trauma, emotionally unavailable parents who are not attuned to the child's needs, or, for the most vulnerable youth, simple uncertainties such as peer teasing or parental discord. Infants who are temperamentally inhibited have higher rates of anxiety disorders in later life. Prospective studies have shown an increased risk of multiple anxiety disorders in middle childhood for children who were classified as behaviorally inhibited as preschoolers.

CLINICAL VIGNETTE

You are called as a consultant to a school to assess Jenn, a 13-year-old eighth-grade girl who has refused to come to school. You find out that Jenn has a long history of multiple absences in school, but this year she came only a few days at the beginning and now is not coming at all. Her mother reports that she has attempted to "drag" her daughter to the car, but Jenn screams and scratches. When she has managed to drive her to school, Jenn will not get out of the car, and even the school social worker and principal cannot persuade her. When you get more history you find that Jenn suffered from separation issues in preschool and kindergarten. The school nurse knows her well, as she visits frequently with complaints of stomachaches and headaches. She refuses to speak in class. She avoids the lunch room and is quiet and nonparticipative in class. Despite this, she had been getting straight A's in school until recently, as not coming to school has negatively impacted her grades. Homework sent to her home is done completely and neatly. Jenn has one friend with whom she spends time. You suspect social anxiety with school phobia. What else should you do? First, talk with the primary care doctor. Chances are the girl has been a frequent visitor there with a variety of somatic complaints. Does she have any medical problems? Try to ascertain if she has been traumatized (bullied, etc.) in school as a reason for her refusal. Get a family history and developmental history from the parents. Discuss the course of the difficulties with the school. Interview Jenn and ask about depressive, anxiety, and psychotic symptoms. If she is suffering from school phobia or social anxiety, consider medication (SSRI), psychotherapy, and an intensive, slow but progressive reintegration into school (often starting with tutoring after school). This is one of the few times that benzodiazepines are indicated in child and adolescent psychiatry. Rapid and effective treatment of the anxiety to help the child be able to get back to school will substantially improve prognosis.

Assessment

When assessing the child or adolescent for whom you suspect an anxiety disorder, it is important to consider other psychiatric disorders, as well as potential for comorbidities (Table 15.1).

TABLE 15.1. Assessment Essentials for Anxiety Disorders

1. Rule out physical causes such as hyperthyroidism, side effects to medications (allergy/asthma medications, etc.), substance abuse, or other medical conditions.
2. Get data from multiple sources. Children are often reluctant to talk about their worries. Be sure to get a family genetic history of anxiety disorders, as well as depression and other mood disorders and tics.
3. Younger children may better communicate their anxieties through drawings or play techniques.
4. Determine the trigger(s) for the anxiety. Does the anxiety only occur in a specific situation? Does it occur "out of the blue"? Does it occur in anticipation of something? Is it pervasive?
5. Understand the environmental and family factors that may affect the youth's anxiety. How do the parents react? Are there family conflicts or other stresses contributing to the anxiety?
6. Screen for comorbid psychiatric disorders: mood disorders, psychosis, eating disorders, tic disorders, and disruptive behavior disorders.
7. Consider the use of symptom rating scales to better categorize, understand, and monitor the child's anxieties. Yale-Brown Obsessive Compulsive Scale (Y-BOCS), the Screen for Child Anxiety Related Emotional Disorders (SCARED), the Social Phobia and Anxiety Inventory for Children (SPAI-C), and the Revised Children's Manifest Anxiety Scale (RCMAS) are suggestions.

Children may suffer from both internalizing and externalizing disorders. Co-occurrence of the inattentive type of ADHD and anxiety disorder is not infrequent. If using a stimulant, "start low and go slow" to minimize the risk of increasing anxiety.

 TIP

Inquire about caffeine intake and counsel to minimize it. Caffeine is a known cause of anxiety.

Treatment

Treatment is multimodal and requires a thoughtful, stepwise intensive treatment of the child and adolescent. Table 15.2 gives the essentials of treatment, elaborating on the types of

TABLE 15.2. Essentials of Multimodal Treatment of Anxiety

1. Psychoeducation of parent and child about the nature of anxiety, how it can affect family relationships, how family members can inadvertently perpetuate the symptoms through their own anxiety, and how the family can support the child in overcoming his or her anxiety.
2. Cognitive-behavioral therapy should comprise first-line treatment. There are evidence-based treatments for OCD (exposure and response prevention), phobias, and other anxiety disorders.
3. School intervention when the anxiety is seriously impairing school functioning.
4. Medications

   1st line: SSRIs—remember that SSRIs can induce anxiety or even panic symptoms in vulnerable individuals so "start low and go slow." Sometimes, benzodiazepines are started concurrently with an SSRI and later tapered once the SSRI confers therapeutic benefits. The SSRIs that are FDA approved for OCD in children include fluoxetine, sertraline, and fluvoxamine (chlomipramine, a TCA, is also approved).

   2nd line: benzodiazepines such as alprazolam, lorazepam, and clonazepam can be useful in the short-term treatment of anxiety, e.g., to reintegrate the child into school. Remember to taper slowly to avoid rebound anxiety.

   3rd line: alpha-2a-agonists—guanfacine and clonidine may be useful for symptoms of hyperautonomic arousal such as palpitations and tachypnea.

   Others: tricyclic antidepressants (TCAs)—requires EKG and blood level monitoring, but may be effective.

   Buspirone—a few case reports of effectiveness in mild anxiety.

   Anticonvulsant agents—case reports for the use of gabapentin, topiramate, and oxcarbazepine. Consider using when other agents have been ineffective.

   Antipsychotic agents—may be useful when all other medications have not been successful or in children with borderline reality testing and high levels of agitation.

---

psychosocial and medication treatment options available. For mild to moderate anxiety, evidence-based psychotherapies and psychoeducation should be used first, with adjunctive medication if necessary. There is evidence that some milder forms of anxiety may have a more prolonged course if medications are started initially. However, for disabling anxiety, consider concomitant psychotherapy and medication.

Anxiety disorders affect a large portion of children and adolescents, causing them tremendous suffering and interfering with optimal development in many domains (social, academic, and life skills). Currently, cognitive behavioral treatments are the best supported interventions and should comprise the first line of treatment. Pharmacotherapy can augment psychosocial treatments individualized to each youth's circumstances and response to psychotherapeutic interventions. Early and effective treatments may improve long-term prognosis.

16 ▼ Early Onset Schizophrenia and Other Psychotic Disorders

Essential Concepts
Screening Questions
- Have you had any experiences like dreaming when you're awake?
- Do you ever hear or see things that other people can't hear or see?
- Do you feel that people are saying bad things about you?
- Do you feel that there is anyone who is out to get you?

A body seriously out of equilibrium, either with itself or with its environment, perishes outright. Not so a mind. Madness and suffering can set themselves no limit.

—George Santayana

CLINICAL DESCRIPTION

Early onset schizophrenia (EOS), with an onset prior to age 18, is an often debilitating disorder characterized by deficits in affect, cognition, and the ability to relate socially with others. This is a rare, but serious disorder, often associated with significant morbidity, chronicity, and psychosocial impairment.

The first important point is that psychosis and schizophrenia are not interchangeable. Psychosis is a general term referring to disordered processing of thoughts and impaired grasp of reality. As such, psychosis or psychotic-like symptoms can occur as a part of many psychiatric syndromes other than schizophrenia, including

- Depression
- Mania
- Schizophreniform disorder
- Psychotic disorder NOS
- Overwhelming stress (brief psychotic disorder)
- Dissociative disorders

- Anxiety disorders (especially PTSD and OCD)
- Substance intoxication or withdrawal
- Personality disorders (PDs)
- Delirium or dementia
- Autistic disorder

Intermittent psychotic symptoms may be frequently observed in children ill enough to require psychiatric hospitalization for a number of disorders. The evaluation of psychotic symptoms in children is complicated as well, as childhood is a natural time for fantasy, imaginary friends, and other illogical thoughts. Differentiating an "overly rich imagination" from a thought disorder may occasionally be difficult. Illogical thinking, social isolation, and inappropriate affect may be seen in autistic disorder, but very early onset, developmental history, and clinical features of lack of social reciprocity as well as the lack of positive symptoms of schizophrenia (such as hallucinations) differentiate the two disorders. Brief psychotic symptoms may be seen during times of stress for a number of children with a variety of vulnerabilities. The symptoms may respond positively to environmental modifications to decrease stress. The take-home point: Evaluate every patient for psychotic symptoms, but don't rush to a diagnosis of early onset schizophrenia.

⊕ KEY POINT

Positive symptoms of schizophrenia include the symptoms that are actively experienced by the individual—florid hallucinations, delusions, and thought disorder. *Negative symptoms* describe a lack of normal experiences, and include flat affect, anergia (lack of energy), and poverty of speech and thought.

In children with early onset schizophrenia (EOS), hallucinations, thought disorder, and flattened affect are the most consistent symptoms (Table 16.1). It is important to distinguish between psychotic thought processes and developmental delays or language disorders.

The types of schizophrenia include paranoid, disorganized, catatonic, undifferentiated, and residual. Schizophreniform disorder includes the same symptoms as schizophrenia, but the episode lasts between 1 and 6 months, whereas schizophrenia lasts for 6 months or more including the prodromal, active, and residual phases. Good prognostic features of schizophreniform disorder are rapid onset of psychotic symptoms,

TABLE 16.1. DSM-IV-TR Criteria for Schizophrenia

Requires two symptoms for 1 month, plus 5 months of prodromal
  or residual symptoms.
Mnemonic: **D**elusions **H**erald **S**chizophrenic's **B**ad **N**ews
Delusions
Hallucinations
Speech disorganization
Behavior disorganization
Negative symptoms (flat affect, paucity of speech, or avolition)

Adapted from American Psychiatric Association (2000), Diagnostic and Statistical Manual of Mental Disorders, 4th ed. Text revision. Washington, DC. American Psychiatric Association.

confusion, good premorbid social and occupational functioning, and absence of blunted or flat affect.

Epidemiology

The usual onset of schizophrenia is late adolescence to early 30s, with men affected on average 5 years earlier than women. It is estimated that 1% of adults suffer from this disorder. Childhood onset schizophrenia is a rare disorder, thought to have a prevalence of 1 to 2 per 1,000. Boys tend to be affected about twice as often as girls. The onset tends to be insidious in most children. There is either a deterioration or failure to reach the expected level of interpersonal, academic, or social achievement. Cognitive functioning tends to be in the low average to average range. Schizophrenia interferes with a child's ability to acquire new information and skills, and he or she tends to fall behind peers academically.

Etiology and Risk Factors

Schizophrenia is a neurobiological illness of complex etiology. As a heterogeneous disorder, no single model of genetic inheritance has been found. It is likely that susceptibility genes act in conjunction with developmental and environmental factors to cause this disorder. Heritability is substantial, with the lifetime risk of developing schizophrenia 10 times higher in first-degree biological relatives of affected individuals when compared to the general population. Other risk factors include obstetrical complications, neurological and seizure disorders, and viral or autoimmune factors.

Neurobiological abnormalities have been found in EOS, including deficits in smooth pursuit eye movements and autonomic responsivity, as well as anatomic and functional changes in brain neuroimaging. Increased ventricular volumes, abnormal hemispheric asymmetries, reduced temporal limbic structure volumes, and abnormal morphology of temporal and frontoparietal cortices have been reported.

We no longer believe that psychological or social factors cause schizophrenia. However, in the context of vulnerability, environmental stress, including high expressed emotion (EE) within the family, may affect the timing, severity, and course of the illness. Thus, psychosocial interventions are critical to prognosis.

KEY POINT

Family high EE has been demonstrated in adult schizophrenic patients to be a risk factor for relapse and poor functioning. EE is the tendency of a family to be highly emotional, loud, and reactive. Family psychoeducation and therapy may improve prognosis by helping family members communicate less emotionally.

CLINICAL VIGNETTE

You are on the Children's Psychiatric Unit of a hospital admitting an 11-year-old boy for threats to kill himself with a knife and then running after his younger brother with a knife threatening to kill him. The boy appears agitated and illogical, although you are finally able to help him calm down and discuss the incident of the day. He reports that his "voices" were telling him to get the knife and "kill." As you get further history, you find that he has never mentioned hallucinations before. He has had episodes of moodiness, threats to kill himself, and socially isolated and irritable behaviors intermittently for several years. You learn that he was started on an antidepressant medication about 3 weeks ago to treat his depression and suicidal thoughts. What further workup is needed to clarify the nature of the psychotic symptoms?

The presentation is likely irritable mania with psychotic features. Hospitalize for safety. Stop the antidepressant medication. Get a medical workup to rule out substance use and thyroid problem, and get general screening labs. Get a more thorough history—talk to outpatient treaters, school, and child and family. Get more thorough family history. Antipsychotic medication may be indicated initially, but you may try to taper after mood stabilizer is at therapeutic level. Discharge planning should consider school, needed intensity of outpatient services, and close medication and safety follow-up.

Assessment

When assessing the child or adolescent for whom you suspect a psychotic disorder or early onset schizophrenia, it is important to consider other psychiatric disorders, as well as potential for comorbidities (Table 16.2).

 TIP

Ask about substance experimentation, and follow up with toxicology screens for all new onset psychosis.

TABLE 16.2. Assessment Essentials for Early Onset Schizophrenia

1. A systematic psychiatric history focusing on a longitudinal understanding of the patient's current and past symptomatology should be obtained.
2. Thorough inquiry about family history of psychiatric disorders and medical illnesses. A cultural history is also needed because cultural and religious beliefs taken out of context may seem psychotic.
3. Multiple informants about child's history and functional level (e.g., child, parents, teachers, past treatment providers) should be included in the evaluation process.
4. Psychoeducational testing is suggested.
5. A comprehensive physical examination is necessary to rule out organic causes of psychotic symptoms. There are no specific laboratory tests, neuroimaging procedures, or other medical workup that is diagnostic. However, EOS is quite rare, and neuroimaging, EEG, and laboratory tests to rule out structural brain abnormalities, seizures, or autoimmune, infectious, thyroid, substance-induced, or other etiologies are often indicated.
6. Younger children may better communicate their psychosis and perceptual disorganization through drawings or play techniques.
7. Baseline and follow-up rating scales that assess positive and negative symptoms and psychosocial functioning are helpful in monitoring the effectiveness of treatment interventions (e.g., Positive and Negative Syndrome Scale for Schizophrenics [PANSS]; Symptom Onset in Schizophrenia [SOS]).

Treatment

Treatment of children with schizophrenia is assumed to be the same treatments that are effective in adults, with modifications for developmental stage and environmental circumstances. A multimodal, multisystems approach that is set up for a long-term course is required. Treatment of nonschizophrenic psychotic disorders requires many of the same services. The medications to treat psychosis are similar, but if the psychosis emanates from a mood or other disorder, antipsychotics may be used adjunctively to treat the psychotic symptoms, but it may not be the mainstay of psychopharmacological treatment. Family therapy and pharmacotherapy combined with social skills training has demonstrated effectiveness in adult patients. Table 16.3 gives the essentials of treatment.

Antipsychotic medications are the foundation for the treatment of psychotic disorders. With childhood-onset schizophrenia, the child will likely require medications for a very

TABLE 16.3. Essentials of Multimodal Treatment of Schizophrenia

1. Psychoeducation of parents and child about the nature of the illness, necessity for treatment compliance, and to provide support and hope for the child and family about the potential to improve with treatment.
2. Psychosocial treatments, including social skills training, supportive psychotherapy, behavior modification, and cognitive-behavioral therapy of dysphoria are all appropriate and should be considered as needed for an individual patient.
3. School interventions may be required to ensure that any special learning needs are addressed. Additionally, children who are quite disabled by the disorders may require special education services and a therapeutic educational program in order to learn.
4. Medications
    1st line: Atypical antipsychotics: risperidone, olanzapine, quetiapine, aripiprazole, ziprasidone
    2nd line: Typical antipsychotics: haloperidol, thiothixene, chlorpromazine, trifluoperazine, molindone
    3rd line: Clozapine, augmentation with lithium or other mood stabilizer, electroconvulsive therapy

Note: Recommendations are drawn from the adult literature and clinical consensus as controlled trials are not yet available justifying the atypical agents as first-line treatments in youth.

prolonged period of time. There is evidence that psychosis left untreated for substantial amounts of time may have a worse prognosis than illness that is treated in its prodromal or early phases. For this reason, judicious use of antipsychotics in a timely manner is recommended. The potential longer-term side effects of the medications (tardive dyskinesia, weight gain or diabetes, cognitive blunting) need to be weighed against the medication effectiveness. Using the smallest amount of medication possible to control the symptoms, exercise and nutrition plan, and close medication monitoring are required. Typical antipsychotics may be as effective as atypical antipsychotics and cause less weight gain. However, dystonias and the potential for tardive dyskinesia and negative symptoms may be of higher risk.

 TIP

Be sure to take a careful assessment of the child's strengths, weaknesses, and environmental resources when devising a treatment plan. Focus on enhancing strengths, while intensively treating the most disabling symptoms.

Eating Disorders: Anorexia Nervosa and Bulimia Nervosa

> **Essential Concepts**
> **Screening Questions**
> - How is your appetite?
> - What do you think about your current weight?
> - When you look in a mirror, what do you think about how you look?
> - Do you ever make yourself throw up after you eat?

CLINICAL DESCRIPTION

Eating disorders in adolescence and young adulthood are quite common, especially in women. Dieting is very frequent, and attempts to be "as thin as possible" may evolve into a serious, disabling, and even life-threatening disorder. An estimated 10% of individuals with serious eating disorders die from complications of the disorder, and another 5% die from suicide.

The two primary eating disorders are anorexia nervosa, with extreme weight loss, and bulimia nervosa, marked by binge eating and often, although not necessarily, with purging (Tables 17.1 and 17.2).

 KEY POINT

Individuals with eating disorders may be secretive about the disorder because they fear intervention or are ashamed. Typically, individuals with anorexia nervosa hide the fact that they are not eating for fear that they will be "forced" to eat more calories. Individuals with bulimia nervosa are often embarrassed about the disorder and will binge in secret. The clinician should always ask about eating and, with adolescents, also ask the family about their observations of a change in eating patterns or weight. Approximately 10 to 15% of eating-disordered individuals are male, with an especially high prevalence in gay men. Therefore, screening questions for eating disorders should be included in all interviews.

TABLE 17.1. DSM-IV-TR Criteria for Anorexia Nervosa

Mnemonic: **W**eight **F**ear **B**others **A**norexics
Refusal to maintain body **W**eight above 85% of expected weight
Intense **F**ear of gaining weight or becoming fat
Distorted **B**ody image
For women: **A**menorrhea (the absence of at least three menstrual
  cycles)
Types: Restricting type or binge-eating/purging type

Adapted from American Psychiatric Association (2000), Diagnostic and Statistical Manual of Mental Disorders, 4th ed. Text revision. Washington, DC. American Psychiatric Association.

Epidemiology

Among women, the lifetime prevalence of anorexia nervosa is 0.5 to 1% and of bulimia nervosa about 4%. Most commonly, the disorder starts in adolescence, often precipitated by a stressful life event. When anorexia nervosa occurs in prepubertal children, it tends to be part of more severe psychopathology, but it is also more likely to resolve. Females are affected 10 times more often than males. The eating disorders tend to be diseases of Westernized countries. In the United States, Whites are more often affected than African Americans or Hispanic Americans.

Etiology and Risk Factors

A combination of biologic, psychological, environmental, and social factors has been implicated in the pathogenesis of eating disorders. Both anorexia and bulimia nervosa are more

TABLE 17.2. DSM-IV-TR Criteria for Bulimia Nervosa

Mnemonic: **B**ulimics **O**ver-**C**onsume **P**astries
Recurrent episodes of **B**inge eating (at least twice a week for
  3 months) that feel **O**ut of control
Excessive **C**oncern with body shape and weight
Purging behaviors, such as self-induced vomiting; misuse of laxatives,
  diuretics, enemas, or other medications; fasting; excessive exercise
Types: Purging type or nonpurging type

Adapted from American Psychiatric Association (2000), Diagnostic and Statistical Manual of Mental Disorders, 4th ed. Text revision. Washington, DC. American Psychiatric Association.

common in high-risk groups that require highly focused attention on weight and appearance, such as ballet, ice-skating, and other sports. High achieving, perfectionistic, competitive individuals with underlying low self-esteem tend to be more commonly affected. Mood disorders, anxiety disorders, substance use, and personality disorders tend to be common comorbidities. Individuals with anorexia nervosa tend to be exquisitely sensitive to perceived rejection, hostility, and conflict. From a family theory perspective, anorexic families often present a conflict-free exterior. This façade is thought to mask a lack of intimacy, enmeshment, rigidity, and conflict. The symptoms of anorexia are thought to focus the family away from the conflict and thus maintain family "homeostasis." In fact, once a pattern of disordered eating begins, multidetermined factors maintain and promote the dysregulated eating patterns. These may include stabilization of the family, binding of anxiety and dsysphoria, and positive reinforcement emanating from compliments about weight loss that may be received from coaches or friends.

🔵 KEY POINT

Severe eating disorders are among the most challenging disorders to treat. Engagement of the patient may be very difficult, as he or she often does not want to gain weight and will engage in increasingly secretive and deceptive maneuvers to avoid taking in calories. I have seen girls sew lead weights into their underclothing prior to being weighed to avoid their weight loss being detected. This lack of joint and collaborative vision of treatment is one of the most difficult aspects of the disorder. Sensitivity and empathy for the patient, along with steadfast adherence to basic physical safety guidelines, are the cornerstones of all treatment.

🔻 TIP

Although eating-disordered patients may be furious about the limits placed in the course of treatment, they are also often relieved that there is external control at a time when they feel out of control.

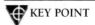**KEY POINT**

Body mass index (BMI: kg/m²) is used to indicate the degree of severity of anorexia nervosa in an individual. A BMI of 17.5 kg/m² correlates with a body weight of less than 85% of the expected.

Assessment

When assessing the child or adolescent for whom you suspect an eating disorder, it is important to ensure an appropriate medical workup and to consider comorbidities, which tend to be common (Table 17.3).

TABLE 17.3. Assessment Essentials for Eating Disorders

1. A comprehensive physical examination is necessary to rule out organic causes of anorexia. Additionally, the physical examination and laboratory assessment should screen for malnutrition and substance use. Anorexia nervosa may present with cachexia, dry skin, lanugo, bradycardia and hypotension, amenorrhea, mild anemia, low serum albumen, and a variety of other abnormalities depending on the degree of cachexia. Bulimia nervosa may present with decreased gag reflex, moth eaten or rough teeth, hypertrophy of the parotids, and electrolyte imbalances.
2. Historic data should be collected from multiple sources. Expect the eating-disordered youth to minimize his or her symptoms and the parents to have significant gaps in their observations of pathologic eating patterns.
3. Psychiatric comorbidity should be identified because eating-disordered patients commonly suffer from comorbid depressive disorders, substance abuse, anxiety disorders, and personality disorders.
4. Family dynamics should be assessed because eating-disordered behaviors tend to exacerbate pathologic family interactions, and such interactions impede recovery.
5. Screening tools such as the "SCOFF" or the Eating Disorders Diagnostic Scale questions may be useful in identifying eating-disordered youths when reviewing mental health status.

TIP

Ask about substance experimentation and follow up with toxicology screens for all bulimia patients. If suspected, screening for laxative and diuretic use is also advised.

CLINICAL VIGNETTE

You are asked to evaluate a 17-year-old junior in high school in late spring. She has been diagnosed with ulcerative colitis, which has been stable for the past 6 months. Despite the fact that her medical condition has stabilized, she has demonstrated ongoing weight loss and dysphoria. Upon meeting, you note that she tends to minimize the effect of her medical issues on her life, and to be quite unconcerned about her recent 18-lb weight loss. She is dressed in baggy sweatshirt and baggy sweat pants, and appears quite cachectic. She denies restricting her food intake, stating that she is just "not hungry." She is quite happy that she does not presently require steroids, as they "made me fat." She has joined the cross-country team and runs at least 4 miles daily. You highly suspect anorexia nervosa, which had its onset with the stress of the medical issues and the weight gain associated with prednisone for her colitis. Her family, with high achieving, intense parents, had not noted how significant her weight loss was until it was brought to their attention in a follow-up visit with the gastroenterologist. The girl states that she is "fine" and tells her parents she does not need a "shrink"; she doesn't know why they even brought her to one. She is medically at a BMI of 17.3 kg/m^2 and is determined to be safe for outpatient treatment. You recommend an intensive program of outpatient psychotherapy, family therapy, weekly weights, and close medical follow-up. You consider a trial of fluoxetine for treatment of obsessionality and depression.

Treatment

Treatment of children and adolescents with eating disorders is assumed to be the same treatment that is effective in adults, with modifications for developmental stage and environmental circumstances. In general, family engagement and family therapy are cornerstones of treatment. No specific medications target eating disorder per se. For that reason, using medications only as needed for specific target symptoms and comorbidity is advised. Table 17.4 gives the essentials of treatment.

TABLE 17.4. Essentials of Multimodal Treatment of Eating Disorders

1. Psychoeducation of parents and youth about the nature of the illness and the necessity of intensive treatment.
2. Determine level of care (inpatient, residential, partial hospital, intensive outpatient, or regular outpatient treatment) that is appropriate depending on the severity of the disorder and medical compromise.
3. Set behavioral goals for improving medical and nutritional status.
4. Reestablish eating as a process based on hunger and satiety cues as well as nourishment needs (e.g., meal support therapy [MST]).
5. Family therapy with a focus on decreasing enmeshment and parental control while facilitating the youth's individuation and minimizing dynamics that promote disordered eating.
6. Developing the patient's and family's tolerance for negative emotions, including the use of anxiety management skills.
7. Supportive psychotherapy, rapport and trust-building, and cognitive-behavioral treatment to help develop adaptive cognitive techniques for addressing the distortions regarding weight and body image.
8. Specific skills building regarding development of a balanced lifestyle, including work, play, and social relationships.
9. School interventions may be required to ensure that the patient is able to maintain appropriate academic progress, while decreasing excessive anxiety and hours of perfectionistic re-doing of homework. The school nurse and mental health professionals in the school need to be aware of and follow any treatment plans.
10. Medications—there are no medications specifically targeting eating disorders.

    1st line: Selective serotonin reuptake inhibitors. For treatment of obsessionality, depression; may help in reducing risk of relapse.

    2nd line: Atypical antipsychotics: risperidone, olanzapine. May be used to facilitate weight gain in anorexic patients by reducing anxiety and thought distortions and increasing appetite.

    Other medications as appropriate for targeted symptoms and comorbid conditions.

(Continued)

TABLE 17.4. **Essentials of Multimodal Treatment of Eating Disorders** (*continued*)

Note: Recommendations are primarily drawn from the adult literature, as there are few controlled trials with adolescents. In general, medication is used for specific target symptoms and comorbidities. Start low and go slow, and monitor vital signs and electrocardiograms.

 TIP

Patients with eating disorders are often quite reassuring to their therapist that they are okay and have their eating issues under control. Be sure to not fall into the trap of agreeing with the patient in minimizing serious symptoms. Although inpatient treatment of eating disorders is becoming less common, ongoing weight loss in the face of medical compromise requires intensive medical and psychiatric stabilization (often on medical floors or combined medical/psychiatric units).

Substance Use Disorders

Essential Concepts
Screening Questions
- Do you smoke cigarettes?
- How often do you drink?
- Do you use any recreational drugs, such as marijuana, LSD, or cocaine?

First you take a drink, then the drink takes a drink, then the drink takes you.

—F. Scott Fitzgerald

CLINICAL DESCRIPTION

Substance use disorders (SUDs) are among the most prevalent psychiatric disorders in young people. Although experimentation with alcohol and drugs is sometimes considered one of the rites of passage for American youth, there is a high risk for misuse, addiction, and serious negative consequences (legal, social, and safety). Additionally, the treatment of any other psychiatric disorders is complicated by concomitant substance use. See Table 18.1 for diagnostic criteria for substance abuse.

Compared to adults, adolescents with SUDs present with a greater number of drugs used at any time. While substance-dependent youth may present with symptoms of tolerance, they present less often with symptoms of withdrawal or other symptoms of dependence noted in Table 18.2.

In general, substance abuse is a disorder that starts in adolescence or early adulthood. In evaluating even a prepubertal child, however, you have a goal to understand if smoking or substance use is present, to understand the nature and severity, and to ensure that it is addressed in treatment. Minors tend to have a higher rate of risk-taking behaviors than adults. They may begin to steal, lie, and participate in criminal behavior to support a habit. SUD youth often have comorbid conduct disorders.

TABLE 18.1. DSM-IV-TR Criteria for Alcohol/Substance Abuse

A maladaptive pattern of alcohol/substance use leading to clinically significant impairment or distress, as manifested by at least one of the following:
1. Failure to fulfill major role obligations at work, school, or home
2. Recurrent alcohol use in situations in which it is physically hazardous
3. Recurrent alcohol-related legal problems
4. Continued alcohol use despite persistent problems caused by its use

Adapted from American Psychiatric Association (2000), Diagnostic and Statistical Manual of Mental Disorders, 4th ed. Text revision. Washington, DC. American Psychiatric Association.

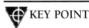 KEY POINT

Youth don't tend to tell parents or other adults about their experimentation with substances. The first clues may be a decline in grades, irritability, or hanging out with a different group of friends. Ask about that.

TABLE 18.2. DSM-IV-TR Criteria for Alcohol/Substance Dependence

Mnemonic: **T**empted **W**ith **C**ognac. To be considered alcohol (or other substance) dependent, the patient must meet at least three of the following seven criteria:

Tolerance—a need for increasing amounts of alcohol to achieve intoxication

Withdrawal syndrome

Loss of **C**ontrol of alcohol use (five criteria follow):
  More alcohol ingested than the patient intended
  Unsuccessful attempts to cut down
  Much time spent in activities related to obtaining or recovering from the effects of alcohol
  Important social, occupational, or recreational activities given up or reduced because of alcohol use
  Alcohol use continued despite the patient's knowledge of significant physical or psychological problems caused by its use

Adapted from American Psychiatric Association (2000), Diagnostic and Statistical Manual of Mental Disorders, 4th ed. Text revision. Washington, DC. American Psychiatric Association.

TIP

Although education about the dangers of substance use is important, it does little to dissuade youth, for whom worries of failing health seem light-years away, from experimenting. Providing alternatives, such as sports or other interests, alcohol-free parties, and other supervised activities is more effective at preventing use.

Epidemiology

It is estimated that over 5 million youth, by age 16, have met the diagnostic criteria for a SUD. In 2003, SUDs were second only to disruptive behavior disorders as the most commonly diagnosed psychiatric disorders in youth—an estimated 12.2% by age 16. In general, boys outnumber girls in rate of substance use. By age 16, 14% of boys and 10% of girls will have experienced an episode of SUD. Tobacco, alcohol, and marijuana are the most commonly used drugs. Almost half of all 12th graders in a recent National Institute of Drug Abuse survey used alcohol within the past month, and around a quarter smoked cigarettes or marijuana. Amphetamines were the second most commonly abused illicit substance, with use by about 5% of high school students. Other substances were less frequently used. By 12th grade, 4% of youth have used anabolic steroids at least once.

Etiology and Risk Factors

There is a complicated and multifactorial set of risk factors for substance abuse (Table 18.3). Alcoholism is the most thoroughly studied of the SUDs. It has a fairly significant genetic vulnerability, with up to 25% of fathers or brothers of an alcoholic individual also suffering from alcoholism. Children of parents with SUDs who are adopted at birth to nondrug-using families have a higher rate of developing SUD than does the general population. Ineffective parenting and inadequate nurturing also increase the risk for developing a SUD. Poor parental supervision and perceived parental approval (or lack of disapproval) of drug use also increase risk.

TABLE 18.3. **Risk Factors for Substance Use Disorders**

- Chaotic home environment
- Parental substance abuse
- Parental mental illness
- Ineffective parenting
- Lack of parental involvement
- Failing school performance
- Poor social coping skills
- Association with conduct-disordered peers
- Perceived parental/peer/community approval of drug use

 KEY POINT

Individuals have the highest risk for continuous lifelong problems with substances if they started using them before the age of 15 years. Marijuana tends to be a "gateway drug" with marijuana use preceding that of cocaine, hallucinogens, and other dangerous substances. However, most marijuana users do not go on to use other substances. With the exceptions of cocaine and prescription drugs, most drug use tends to decrease after the age of 25.

Assessment

When assessing the child or adolescent for whom you suspect a substance use disorder, it is important to ensure an appropriate medical workup and to consider comorbidities, which tend to be common (Table 18.4).

CLINICAL VIGNETTE

This is an excerpt from an interview of a 16-year-old young man whom a resident is evaluating in outpatient clinic for a change in his behavior—he has become quite irritable and defiant of rules, his grades are slipping, and he has started staying out past curfew at night. His parents and teachers suspect that he has started using substances, but he has denied it. When the resident meets him, the youth is charming, engaging, and cooperative.

Interviewer: *You seem to be a popular guy.*
Youth: *Sort of, I guess.*

TABLE 18.4. Assessment Essentials for Substance Use Disorders

1. A comprehensive physical examination, with screening laboratory tests, including liver function tests, blood count, and toxicology (drug) screen.
2. Historic data should be collected from multiple sources (patient, parents, siblings, teachers, caseworkers, and peers, if possible). The patient alone is likely to minimize or deny use.
3. Try to determine how many psychoactive substances are being used and how available they are. Where and with whom is he or she using?
4. Determine if the youth has drug use, abuse, or dependence.
5. Assess family and home situation. How closely is the youth supervised? What is the overall communication level, involvement, and home support for the youth?
6. Obtain a genetic family history of substance abuse as well as alcohol and substance use by members of the family in the home.
7. Assess for other psychiatric comorbidity.
8. Substance abuse rating instruments can be helpful in screening for SUDs and for monitoring treatment response (e.g., **S**ubstance-**A**buse **S**ubtle **S**creening **I**nventory [SASSI]; **P**ersonal **E**xperience **S**creening **Q**uestionnaire [PESQ]; **A**dolescent **D**iagnostic **I**nterview [ADI]).

   Another screening tool normed for individuals over 16 is the CAGE Questionnaire—a mnemonic for attempts to *cut* back on drinking, being *annoyed* at criticisms about drinking, feeling *guilty* about drinking, and using alcohol as an *eye* opener).

Interviewer:	*Do you and your friends smoke when you hang out together?*
Youth:	*Sometimes.*
Interviewer:	*Get invited to parties?*
Youth:	*Yeah, some.*
Interviewer:	*Besides alcohol, what is available at the parties?*
Youth:	*Just a little weed.*

From there, the resident has set the stage for the expectation of alcohol and drugs to be at parties, and assuming he may be experimenting with them. She can then get to know more details about the drugs available and which ones this young man is using.

TIP

A word about confidentiality: Just as suicidal risk cannot be kept confidential, neither should dangerous substance abuse or dependence. Be sure that you don't tell the youth that all of the information he tells you is confidential, such that you are in a dilemma if you find out about substance abuse. Instead, let him know that you will support him in telling his parents if there is something that puts him at risk that they need to know.

Treatment

Treatment of children and adolescents with substance use disorders is multimodal and family centered (Table 18.5). No specific medications have demonstrated effectiveness in children and adolescents at curbing drug craving. The youth should stop using substances and be reassessed for psychiatric comorbidity prior to starting a medication to target symptoms of the comorbidity. Effective treatment of ADHD may decrease the risk of substance abuse.

TABLE 18.5. Essentials of Multimodal Treatment of Substance Use Disorders

1. Psychoeducation of parents and youth about the nature of the illness (including relapsing nature of SUDs) and the necessity of treatment.
2. Family therapy and involvement are critical to treatment. Improving communication is the primary focus. Additionally, addressing issues such as lack of parental involvement in the child's life, the need for clear family rules, and untreated parental SUDs may be targeted. Multisystemic therapy (MST) may focus on removing the youth from environments that trigger the use.
3. Set up a plan to avoid situations that trigger substance use (such as friends or hangouts).
4. Cognitive behavior therapy may be used to target thinking errors associated with substance abuse and to increase self control.
5. Group therapies and 12-step approaches may be helpful. Beware of the risk of "peer deviancy training" in groups with conduct disorders, in which younger, more naïve members learn "bad habits" from other group members.

(Continued)

TABLE 18.5. Essentials of Multimodal Treatment of Substance Use Disorders (*continued*)

6. Inpatient rehabilitation may be required for drug dependence. Intensive outpatient services are also indicated for the more seriously impaired youth.

7. School interventions may be required to ensure that the youth is receiving the services required to help motivate and engage him or her in the academic process. School counseling is often indicated.

8. There are medications aimed at treating intoxication states and withdrawal conditions, preventing continued use, and providing narcotic maintenance (e.g., naltrexone, disulfiram, methadone for heroin addiction, and benzodiazepines for withdrawal states). In general, substance abuse treatment tends to minimize psychotropic medication use. To fully assess psychiatric comorbidities, the substance use disorder must have been addressed. However, medication may be indicated for comorbidities.

   ADHD comorbidity: Substance abuse has been demonstrated to be lower when ADHD is effectively treated. Atomoxetine, bupropion, or guanfacine may be indicated first-line. The long-acting stimulant medications (that cannot be crushed and snorted) may also be used carefully in an at-risk population if the medication administration is closely monitored.

   Use other medications as appropriate for targeted symptoms and comorbid conditions.

   In general, it is advised that a youth be observed for several weeks off substances to determine whether another psychiatric condition persists prior to starting a medication.

✦ KEY POINT

One of the best deterrents to substance abuse in teens is open communication at home. Parents who confront their teen if they suspect substance use, let him or her know that they do not condone it, and provide a safe environment in which to disclose his or her use and get help with abstinence tend to have briefer and less severe periods of use and to have better long-term prognosis.

Trauma-Related Disorders

All children have to be deceived if they are to grow up without trauma.

—Kazuo Ishiguro

CLINICAL DESCRIPTION

Many children grow up with the scars of physical or sexual abuse, domestic violence, or other traumas. Natural disasters, war, and serious illness with painful procedures are other sources of trauma. It is impossible to grow up without some bad things happening. However, for some children, the horrors they have had to endure have left serious emotional scars.

Posttraumatic stress disorder (PTSD) is an emotional disorder that occurs following an overwhelming and frightening event that threatened serious bodily harm. It results in a re-experiencing of the traumatic event and avoidance of situations that activate traumatic memories. In infants and young children, neglect or maltreatment may result in emotional consequences as well (Table 19.1). Reactive attachment disorder (RAD) is characterized by disturbed and distrusting social relatedness caused by grossly pathogenic care. This disorder results in the child displaying severe inhibition and hypervigilance in social interactions (inhibited type) or indiscriminate attachment and familiarity with any adult who is nice to them (disinhibited type). Children who are traumatized often are quite reactive and stress sensitive, tend to perceive the world as a dangerous place, and tend to interpret other people's behavior as menacing or aggressive.

TABLE 19.1. DSM-IV-TR Criteria for Posttraumatic Stress Disorder

Trauma exposure	The child has been exposed to an event that involved threatened death or serious injury to him/herself or others. The child's response to the trauma was expressed by disorganized or agitated behavior (or intense fear, helplessness, and horror).
Trauma re-experience (1 or more)	Repetitive play of trauma themes in young children. Recurrent intrusive distressing recollections of the event (images, thoughts, or perceptions) for others. Frightening dreams or recurrent dreams of the event. Trauma-specific reenactment in young children. Acting or feeling like the traumatic event was recurring, e.g., flashbacks. Intense psychological distress or physiological reactivity on exposure to something that resembles the traumatic event.
Trauma avoidance (3 or more)	Efforts to avoid thoughts, feelings, activities that prompt recollection of the trauma. Inability to recall aspects of the trauma. Diminished interest or feelings of detachment. Restricted range of affect. Sense of foreshortened future.
Increased arousal (2 or more)	Difficulty falling or staying asleep. Irritability or outbursts of anger. Difficulty concentrating. Hypervigilance and/or exaggerated startle response.

Adapted from American Psychiatric Association (2000), Diagnostic and Statistical Manual of Mental Disorders, 4th ed. Text revision. Washington, DC. American Psychiatric Association.

CLINICAL VIGNETTE

Sylvia is a 5-year-old girl who was adopted from an orphanage in Europe at the age of 3. Her biological parents were both substance abusers, and Sylvia had lived on the streets with them, exposed to neglect and unknown traumas, until she was 2, at which time she arrived at the orphanage, poorly nourished and "famished." Sylvia quickly made friends at the orphanage, calling all of the women who worked there "Mama." When she was adopted by parents from the United States, she called her new mother "Mama" right away and seemed to attach immediately. Sylvia has been well cared for by her parents and has been in very good day-care when her parents are at work. Difficulties with severe temper tantrums when she does not get her way prompted the day-care provider to suggest referral. When you meet her, Sylvia is a beautiful, blue-eyed girl who immediately takes your hand to walk to your office. She is chatty and has mild articulation errors, but otherwise seems to be developing well. You play together, and she directs the action of dolls in the dollhouse repeatedly being attacked by "burglars". When it gets time for her to leave your office and the toys with which you have been playing, she begins to pout, cry, and refuse to go with her mother. You are concerned about Sylvia's trauma history and her symptoms of RAD, disinhibited type.

 KEY POINT

PTSD is only one of several diagnosable psychiatric disorders that may emerge from trauma. Depression, other anxiety disorders, substance abuse, conduct problems, and (in infancy) reactive attachment disorder are others. Screen for these, as well.

 KEY POINT

Exposure to violence during childhood often negatively impacts development in multiple domains. Be attentive to neurophysiological signs (stress response, startle and hyperarousal reactions, dissociation), altered cognitions (feeling vulnerable, sense of foreshortened future, lowered self-confidence, and guilt), and emotional development (core identity, view of the world, social relationships). All aspects of the child's development may be impacted.

Epidemiology

Trauma is a common occurrence in our communities. The National Center on Child Abuse and Neglect reported in 2000 that over 3 million children per year are referred to child protective services for abuse or serious neglect. One-third of these cases are substantiated and half of these (over half a million) are so severe that the children are removed from their homes. Community violence, domestic violence, natural disasters, accidents, and other events may be so severe as to leave permanent scars on the child's developing personality. In inner cities, children may be exposed to shootings or stabbings (up to 40% according to Schwab-Stone). September 11th was a national trauma, which affected children in the vicinity much more intensely.

It appears that children are more sensitive to the effects of trauma than adults and consequently may exhibit higher rates of PTSD development. Community-based studies reveal a lifetime prevalence for PTSD of approximately 8% of the adult population in the United States.

Etiology and Risk Factors

The etiology of PTSD requires an overwhelming stressful event. However, not all individuals who experience severe trauma develop a disorder. Clearly, there is a complex interplay between the environmental event, the person's premorbid psychological health and psychosocial support network, and a neurobiological cascade that characterizes the pathogenesis.

One important factor is whether the trauma was a single event or multiple events. Children's symptoms also vary as a function of age and developmental phase. Single-incident trauma can have a profound and long-lasting effect. Half of victims generally recover within 3 months, but many remain ill for a year or more, with symptoms reemerging following a subsequent trauma or life stress. Complex trauma consists of multiple exposures to stressful events over time. There is an estimated 37.5% lifetime prevalence for PTSD in victims of substantiated childhood abuse and neglect. Chronic trauma adversely affects personality development. Symptoms of chronic trauma are impairment of affect regulation, chronic destructive behavior to self and others, dissociation, and problems with attention and somatization. The individual may suffer from brief psychotic symptoms.

Early life trauma affects multiple neurobiological functions. Dysregulation of the hypothalamic-pituitary-adrenal (HPA) axis and the secretion of the stress hormone cortisol are noted in children and adults. Maltreated children have shown overall smaller cerebral volumes, with normal hippocampal size, in neuroimaging studies. Multiple neurotransmitters have been implicated in the traumatic stress response as well. It is clear that severe stress leads to global dysregulation (neuroendocrine, biological, psychological, and developmental) and the high potential for longer-term emotional and behavioral sequellae.

Assessment

When assessing the child or adolescent for whom you suspect abuse, neglect, or there is a known trauma, it is important to ensure an appropriate medical workup and to consider comorbidities, which tend to be common (Table 19.2).

TABLE 19.2. Essentials for Assessment of Trauma in Children

1. A comprehensive physical examination, with screening for physical injury or sexual abuse, as appropriate.
2. Historic data should be collected from multiple sources regarding the trauma (or suspected trauma) and the child's symptoms.
3. Forming a rapport and providing a safe environment in which to assess the child are critical.
4. Ask direct questions about the trauma of the traumatized children.
5. If a child is reluctant to talk directly about the trauma (or developmentally would not be expected to do so), help the child communicate his or her inner life experience through nonverbal methods, e.g., play or artwork.
6. Assess family and home situation. Is it a safe environment for the child? Are protective services involved (or do they need to be)? Was the entire family traumatized? What supports does the family require to provide for the traumatized child?
7. Assess for psychiatric comorbidity.
8. Structured rating instruments may be helpful as one component of a comprehensive evaluation (e.g., Trauma Symptom Checklist for Children [TSCC]; Child Posttraumatic Stress Reaction Index [CPTS-RI]).

CLINICAL VIGNETTE

This is an excerpt from an interview of a 6-year-old girl who was in a car accident in which her babysitter, the driver, died. She is in the hospital a week later being treated for a broken leg and cuts. She has been tearful and irritable, and eating poorly. You are a consultant asked to see her around "processing the trauma." You met her one other time, and are back to see her.

Interviewer:	*You were in a very bad accident. Can you tell me about it?*
Sarah:	*It wasn't an accident!*
Interviewer:	*Tell me what you mean.*
Sarah:	*I was mad.*
Interviewer:	*You were mad?*
Sarah:	*Yes! I wanted to go to the store, and she said we had to go home.*
Interviewer:	*And then?*
Sarah:	*I think she'd had it with me.*
Interviewer:	*How do you mean?*
Sarah:	*She said, "No, Sarah. We need to get home today to practice the piano before your lesson." I think she just didn't want to deal with me anymore.*
Interviewer:	*Are you thinking you caused the crash?*
Sarah:	*How else could it have happened?*

Sarah is presenting with classical survivor guilt. She was attempting to resolve in her own mind how this horrible accident could have happened. She has been living with the shame and guilt that she caused the accident, and that her babysitter wanted to "get away" from her. When that was finally talked out, over a period of weeks, her severe dysphoria and irritability began to subside.

 TIP

A word about mandated reporting. All physicians, teachers, and mental health providers are mandated reporters. If there is reason to suspect abuse or neglect, you are mandated to inform your state's protective service agency. There is a hotline and a form to be filled out. If you are treating a child who informs you of being hit with a belt, touched inappropriately, etc., you must file. Unless contraindicated for a specific reason, rapport may be maintained if you talk with the parents or guardians about why you are concerned and inform them that you will be filing a report. You are modeling honesty, openness, and your dedication to the safety of the child.

Treatment

Although much remains to be done, there is an increasing literature on the treatment of trauma in children. A "prevention-intervention" model incorporates triage for children exposed to violence, support and strengthening of coping skills to prepare for anticipated trauma and grief responses, treatment of other disorders that may develop or be exacerbated in the context of PTSD, and treatment of acute PTSD. All humans have the basic need to feel connected and share with others. Providing the time and a format for the child to put experience into words and thus share traumatic events with others in a safe and secure manner can be a potent early intervention. A well-planned treatment typically includes an admixture of cognitive-behavioral, family-supportive, and psychodynamically informed psychotherapy in several phases: initial or preventive therapy, long-term therapy, and pulsed intervention (Tables 19.3 and 19.4). Central to almost all treatment strategies is the emphasis on re-exposing the individual to traumatic cues under safe conditions, and incorporative mastery elements in a structured and supportive manner.

 TIP

Trauma can have negative effects on personality development. Early detection, intervention, and a plan to ensure that the child is safe and the risk of repeated trauma is minimized will most effectively improve prognosis. One of the most satisfying aspects of child psychiatry is the opportunity to prevent disability—treatment of trauma is one of the most important and promising of those opportunities.

TABLE 19.3. Essentials for Treatment of Traumatized Children

1. Initial intervention—debriefing. This is an opportunity for children to share their experiences in a safe and nurturing setting. Critical incident stress debriefing, psychological first aid, or just the opportunity for children to clarify and talk about (or draw or play about) their traumatic experience is the initial intervention. Triage children who display serious symptoms for more intensive treatment.
2. Psychoeducation of parents and children about the components of PTSD and the specific rationale for therapy is critical.
3. The treatment provided may depend on whether there was a shared trauma (such as the 9/11 attacks) or an individual one (such as being a victim of sexual abuse).
4. Psychosocial therapies
   • Group cognitive-behavioral treatment for PTSD (such as that formulated by Amaya-Jackson and colleagues)
   • Trauma-focused cognitive-behavioral therapy (TF-CBT)
   • Brief therapy with controlled exposure to traumatic cues and "working through"
   • Family therapy—to help the family learn coping strategies, increase communication, and help them meet the child's needs adequately
   • Group therapy and shared working through
   • Long-term and intermittent supportive therapy—continuity with the therapist can be very helpful in ongoing working through issues of trauma in a longer-term or intermittent or "pulsed" therapy manner.
5. School interventions may be required to ensure that the youth is receiving the services required to help him or her feel safe and secure in school. School counseling is often indicated.
6. Medications—as an adjunct to treat overwhelming anxiety, facilitate functioning, and help the child to be more amenable to psychotherapy. The decision to use medication is based on target symptoms, their severity, and the degree of disability they cause. Table 19.4 gives the medications that may be effective in the treatment of PTSD.

TABLE 19.4. Medications Used in the Treatment of Posttraumatic Stress Disorder

Medication Category	Examples Commonly Used in Pediatric Populations	Target Symptoms/Comments
Serotonergic agents	Fluoxetine, sertraline, citalopram, nefazodone	Reported to be effective in treating hyperarousal, agitation, and insomnia. Considered a first-line treatment for PTSD.
Alpha-2a agonists	Clonidine, guanfacine	Reported to be effective in treating hyperarousal, agitation, insomnia, and nightmares. Considered a first-line treatment for PTSD.
Beta-blocker	Propranolol	Shown effective for treating target symptoms of hyperarousal and agitation. Considered second line because of problems with side effects, dizziness.
Tricyclic antidepressants	Imipramine, desipramine, nortriptyline	Good for sleep dysregulation and associated enuresis. Considered second line because of the cardiotoxicity side-effect profile.

(Continued)

TABLE 19.4. Medications Used in the Treatment of Posttraumatic Stress Disorder (*continued*)

Medication Category	Examples Commonly Used in Pediatric Populations	Target Symptoms/Comments
Benzodiazepines	Lorazepam, diazepam, clonazepam	Brief use for insomnia. Probably underutilized in children because of worries of abuse or dependence. Short-term use would minimize this risk. Watch for disinhibition. Considered second line by many.
Mood stabilizers	Valproate, carbamazepine, oxcarbazepine	Carbamazepine, shown to be effective in decreasing flashbacks, nightmares, intrusive memories, and sleep dysregulation in children and adults. Considered second line by some because of side-effect profile and the need for blood testing.
Antipsychotics	Risperidone, olanzapine, quetiapine, aripiprazole, ziprasidone, haloperidol	Should be reserved for youth with associated psychotic symptoms, or extreme aggression or self-injurious behaviors.

Reprinted with permission from Cheng & Meyers: *Child and Adolescent Psychiatry: The Essentials*, Lippincott Williams & Wilkins, 2005.

Adjustment Disorders

Essential Concepts
Screening Questions
- Has there been something that happened recently that has caused you to feel particularly upset?
- What was it? When did it happen?
- What type of response have you had to that event?

Every new adjustment is a crisis in self-esteem

—Eric Hoffer

CLINICAL DESCRIPTION

Life is full of events that cause upset and stress. At times a particular stress may precipitate a significant decline in ability to cope. When this happens, a child, adolescent, or adult may experience extreme distress, depression, anxiety, or behavioral symptoms as a consequence. We diagnose an adjustment disorder when the symptoms are not specifically related to bereavement and do not meet criteria for another Axis I or II disorder, but have resulted in significant impairment in functioning within 3 months of the stressor. In children and adolescents, divorce or separation of parents, a move to a new school or home, or being teased at school may result in a distress reaction. When the reaction is excessive and interferes with daily life tasks, it becomes an adjustment disorder.

CLINICAL VIGNETTE

Brittany is a 13-year-old seventh-grade girl presenting with symptoms of anxiety, crying spells, and recent shoplifting, which was quite uncharacteristic, as she was described by her parents as an honor student who had been very well behaved. Her parents have been arguing a great deal, and last month announced to Brittany and her 7-year-old sister that they are divorcing. Her father will be taking a new job and moving 2 hours away. Brittany speaks freely to you and relates that she "had a perfect life, and now it is totally ruined!" She is quite close to her father and feels abandoned by his move. Her parents, although well meaning, tried to shield the issues from the children by stating, "It will all work out." They subtly and not so subtly let the children know that this was not a topic for discussion. Brittany tells you that she has begun to hang out "with other kids from broken homes, since I am one now." The shoplifting and other behaviors are a manifestation of her distress (and possibly an attempt to reunite her family).

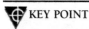 KEY POINT

An adjustment disorder is an appropriate diagnosis to make for a child or adolescent who is responding acutely to a stressor. If the stressor is significant, consider posttraumatic stress disorder (PTSD) as a diagnosis. If there is a more chronic disorder that does not resolve with the resolution of the stress, rethink the diagnosis.

Epidemiology

Adjustment disorders tend to be common. It is estimated that between 2 and 8% of youth in community samples suffer from this disorder. For clinical samples, the rate is higher.

Etiology and Risk Factors

The diagnosis of adjustment disorder assumes a stressor. However, as with PTSD, some children and adolescents respond more negatively to stress than others. There are important intrinsic factors that modulate the impact of a distressing event. Cognitive and emotional development and pre-stress self-esteem and level of psychosocial support all mediate the reaction the child has to the stress. Because children often link unrelated events as cause-and-effect phenomena, they may feel guilt and distress over uncontrollable events that they did not cause.

TIP

Children with chronic illnesses will often meet criteria for an adjustment disorder. New diagnoses of juvenile diabetes or epilepsy commonly lead to adjustment difficulties. The child and family need a great deal of support to prevent more significant and permanent psychiatric disability.

Assessment

The primary issue in assessment is determining if there is a pre-existing psychiatric disorder that has been exacerbated by stress, or if the stress reaction constitutes PTSD, a major depressive episode, or other psychiatric disorder.

Treatment

Treatment of children and adolescents with adjustment disorders is focused on two primary issues—resolving the acute stressor and shoring up coping mechanisms. Family intervention is typically the treatment of choice—helping the family cope with the stress, helping the family support the child, and decreasing the "sick role" labeling of the child.

Psychoeducation of children, adolescents, and families about reactions to stress is the first aspect of treatment. Supportive psychotherapy, family counseling, and brief, focused treatment of the presenting symptoms are indicated. Pharmacological treatment to target the child's reactive symptoms and alleviate immediate stress may be useful in specific situations. In general, there is very little research around the efficacy of medications for the treatment of adjustment disorder.

CLINICAL VIGNETTE

Sharelle is a 10-year-old girl who tends to be a perfectionist and does very well in school. There is a strong family history of anxiety disorders and obsessive-compulsive personality in her biological father and grandfather. Sharelle had no significant symptoms until approximately 1 month ago, when she was at a sleepover at a friend's home and became ill in the night (vomiting). She now presents a month later, fearful of going to school for fear of the humiliation of vomiting in public. In fact, it has been a week since spring break (a week of school vacation) and she has only gone to school once. When she got to school, she went immediately to the nurse stating she was ill and needed to go home. She has started eating less and is losing weight. You diagnose an adjustment disorder and begin psychoeducation, supportive psychotherapy, relaxation treatment, and medication to target her phobic reaction to going to school. With some low-dose benzodiazepines and the psychosocial treatments, she is able to get back to school. Ongoing anxiety symptoms (continued preoccupation about vomiting) suggest that she may require a longer-term treatment with an SSRI and cognitive-behavioral therapy as well. In this case, the stressor (vomiting) may be the first symptom of the onset of a longer-term anxiety disorder.

SPECIAL CLINICAL
CIRCUMSTANCES

Psychiatric Emergencies in Child and Adolescent Psychiatry

Essential Concepts

- The top priority is to minimize the acute risk of the child or adolescent causing harm to himself or others.
- Ask the child or adolescent directly about suicidal and homicidal thoughts and intent.
- The youth may minimize risk of dangerousness. Be sure to get history from multiple sources in your assessment.
- Is there concurrent substance use?
- Is there an acute psychiatric disorder that requires treatment, such as psychotic or manic symptoms?

CLINICAL DESCRIPTION

The suffering of children and youth in the throes of a psychiatric emergency is palpable. They frequently feel desperate and hopeless. Suicidal ideation, suicide attempt, or seriously out of control behavior are the most common child and adolescent psychiatric emergencies and will be the focus of the chapter (Table 21.1).

In assessing children and youth in crisis, you are faced with the difficult decision regarding the management of these patients, such as when to recommend (or require) hospitalization, how to facilitate acute outpatient treatment, dealing with recurrent suicide attempts, and ameliorating the social chaos that often surrounds these youth. These decisions are taxing even for experienced physicians. Assessing and providing stabilization for youth in psychiatric crisis are critical skills for all child and adolescent psychiatrists (Table 21.2).

TABLE 21.1. **Types of Psychiatric Emergencies for Children and Adolescents**

Suicidal ideation, intent, gesture, or attempt
Serious aggression toward others or threats of violence (including firesetting or sexual perpetration)
Psychosis or mania
Acute anxiety or panic
Conversion symptoms
Anorexia nervosa or bulimia nervosa
Running away or high-risk behaviors
Delirium or acute mental status change
Substance abuse
Victim of physical or sexual assault or abuse
Acute school refusal

TABLE 21.2. **Essential Emergency Child and Adolescent Psychiatric Assessment**

1. Rule out an acute medical issue (such as overdose, intoxication, head trauma, or other).
2. Demographics—age, residence, caretakers.
3. Presenting complaint—details of the events that precipitated the crisis assessment.
4. History of present illness—symptoms have presented for how long? How severe? Acute stressors. Get information from multiple sources (youth, parent/guardian, teachers or others, as appropriate).
5. Psychiatric history—prior treatment, taking medications, psychiatric symptoms (depression, suicide attempts, psychosis, aggression, substance abuse).
6. Risk assessment—suicidal thoughts, prior attempts, intent, what means, physical or sexual abuse, recent stressors, access to means (firearms, medication, etc.), homicidal thoughts, revenge fantasies, level of impulse control.
7. Developmental history—learning issues, friends, regression in functioning.
8. Family situation—living situation, communication in the family, abuse, neglect, or substance use in the family, family support, supervision, firearms or other dangers in the home.
9. Family genetic history of psychiatric illness, suicide, incarceration, learning issues.
10. Medical history—current or prior acute or chronic illness, medication.

(Continued)

TABLE 21.2. Essential Emergency Child and Adolescent
Psychiatric Assessment (*continued*)

11. Mental status exam—with focus on thought process, psychosis,
organicity, hopelessness, insight and judgment, motivation for
help, ability to form alliance, acute psychiatric status (review of
psychiatric symptoms, including neurovegetative symptoms,
psychosis, mania, obsessive thoughts, etc.), suicidal thoughts,
and thoughts of revenge.

 KEY POINT

Youth may say that they are "fine" and minimize the risk of
their violent or suicidal behavior once they are calm. You must
check with others to determine how serious the behavior was.
Even if the youth has calmed, if the behavior put him or her
in serious danger, acute treatment in the hospital or other
intensive treatment setting may be required.

 TIP

An emergency evaluation must be brief and focused. Assess
immediately for the acute potential for the child hurting himself or others. Rule out acute intoxication, overdose, or medical illness with a change in mental status (such as delirium
or psychosis). Ensure that the patient is safe and contained
as you get the remainder of the information required.

 KEY POINT

Risk factors are cumulative for predicting suicide. The severity of stressors is also important in predicting suicidal behavior, especially severe acute stressors.

Epidemiology of Suicidality

In the United States, approximately 2 million teenagers attempt
suicide each year, while 2,000 die of suicide. Suicide is the
3rd leading cause of death for those aged 14 to 18, and the

12th leading cause of death among children aged 13 and younger. Firearms are the most common method of suicide, followed by hanging, jumping, carbon monoxide poisoning, and self-poisoning. Firearms are clearly the most lethal method of suicide attempt, being 200 times more likely than drug overdose to end in death. The use of alcohol combined with access to firearms has emerged as the major factor differentiating completed suicides from attempts.

The Centers for Disease Control and Prevention found that 19% of high school students had "seriously considered suicides," with nearly 15% having made a specific plan, 9% having made an attempt, and 2.6% having made a medically serious attempt. Thus, suicidality is of epidemic proportions. Females tend to contemplate suicide or attempt suicide more often, whereas males tend to complete suicide more often, using more lethal means. In males, a history of suicidal behavior increases the risk of completed suicide. In females, the association is present, but not as strong. There was a marked increase in suicide rates in the several decades prior to 1990. The good news is that the numbers of completed suicides in teens has declined over the past decade.

Etiology and Risk Factors

Although the exact etiology of suicide is unknown, multiple risk factors have been identified, as summarized in Table 21.3. Most, although not all, suicidal youth have a major psychiatric disorder—usually a mood disorder, although substance abuse, conduct disorder, and psychosis increase risk as well. Youth who are struggling with issues of sexual orientation may be highly stressed and at increased risk of self-harm.

CLINICAL VIGNETTE

This is an excerpt from an interview of a 16-year-old young woman whom a resident is evaluating in outpatient crisis clinic for suicidality. She told a counselor at school that she wanted to kill herself, and the resident was asked to "clear her" before she was allowed to return to school. Her parents and teachers report that she has seemed depressed and withdrawn over the past month. She broke up with her boyfriend of 6 months the week before. The family is appropriately concerned about her and has been trying to get her in to see a child and adolescent psychiatrist, but the appointment is still another 3 weeks away. When you meet the girl, she appears irritable and dysphoric.

Interviewer:	You told your school counselor that you were feeling suicidal. Tell me about that.
Youth:	What's the use, anyway?
Interviewer:	How long have you been feeling this bad?
Youth:	A very long time. But it got worse when I found out my boyfriend was cheating on me. It seems that I can't trust anyone.
Interviewer:	You must have been very hurt.
Youth:	Yeah, I guess you could say that.
Interviewer:	So hurt you wanted to die?
Youth:	It's not just that. It seems like there is no hope. My grades are slipping. I have disappointed my parents. My best friend moved away last year. I just can't take it anymore.

TABLE 21.3. Essential Risk Factors for Suicidality

1. History of suicidality (past attempts predict future suicidality)
2. Lethality of suicide attempt or intent
3. Psychiatric disorders that fuel suicidality
   - Bipolar disorder
   - Depression
   - Substance abuse
   - Psychosis
   - Conduct disorder, especially impulsive/aggressive
4. Personality traits
   - Impulsivity
   - Aggression
   - Perfectionism/Inflexibility
   - Hopelessness
5. Family factors
   - Parental mood disorders, suicidality, substance abuse
   - Family conflict and poor communication
   - Poor supervision and poor support
6. Acute stressors
   - Loss—romantic, parents, peers, prestige
   - Disciplinary crisis
   - Legal involvement/incarceration
   - School failure
7. Access to means
   - Firearms
   - Other highly lethal means
   - Inadequate supervision

From there, the resident asks more specific questions about suicidal plans, intent, and psychiatric symptoms (neurovegetative symptoms of depression, substance use, psychotic symptoms, etc.). Concern about the level of hopelessness precipitated her admission to an adolescent psychiatric inpatient unit for acute treatment and stabilization.

 TIP

A word about confidentiality: Suicidality and homicidality cannot be kept confidential. If you have reason to believe a child or youth is in danger, you must ensure treatment. Rarely, but occasionally, this may mean involuntary commitment for treatment. A need to notify may be required if the youth is homicidal.

Treatment

Treatment of children and adolescents with acute psychiatric emergencies is multimodal, with the first requirement of ensuring safety. Tables 21.4 and 21.5 provide a treatment decision tree and appropriate treatment interventions for suicidal youth.

TABLE 21.4. Treatment Decision Tree for Suicidal Youth

1. Suicide attempt
   - Emergency room and crisis stabilization
   - Hospitalize on psychiatric unit
2. Suicidal ideation with plan or suicidal ideation with highly lethal thoughts
   - Urgent outpatient psychiatric assessment if interim safety can be ensured
   - Parents must agree to supervise adequately and to secure lethal means of self-harm in home while awaiting urgent outpatient assessment
   - Emergency room evaluation if interim safety cannot be ensured
3. Suicidal ideation without a plan
   - Routine psychiatric assessment if within reasonable time, if parental supervision is adequate, and if removal of means of self-harm ensured
   - Urgent psychiatric assessment if due to exacerbated psychiatric disorder, or if routine appointment not readily available, or if parent cannot adequately supervise or secure means of self-harm

TABLE 21.5. Treatment Essentials for Suicidal Youth

1. Identification and development of a continuum of interventions, including use of emergency room, crisis services, inpatient unit, outpatient services, "wrap around" services, and respite care
2. Development of a treatment team that includes various providers: primary care provider, primary mental health clinician and/or child and adolescent psychiatrist, school counselor, and other clinicians as needed and available
3. Active diagnosis and aggressive treatment of psychiatric illness
4. Individual therapies emphasizing the development of problem-solving skills and impulse control, cognitive-behavioral therapies, and dialectic behavioral therapy, as appropriate
5. Family interventions, emphasizing the development of nonviolent conflict resolution and enhanced communication skills
6. "Harm reduction" through modifications of stressful life obligations such as school schedule
7. Development of family and community resources; emphasize community supports for youth with psychiatrically compromised parents or from unsupportive homes

 KEY POINT

Suicide prevention strategies include those designed to increase recognition of youth at risk and facilitate referral to mental health services, as well as those designed to address risk factors. Education, screening, peer support programs, school and community gatekeeper training, crisis services/hotlines, and interventions after a suicide to prevent "contagion" are current methods used to decrease the risk of suicide in the population.

 TIP

Ask what the youth aspires to do. If he or she is forward thinking, that is a good prognostic sign.

 TIP

Recently devised youth self-report scales for assessing suicidality which may be useful include the Columbia Suicide Screen

(CSS), Reasons for Living Inventory for Adolescents (RFL-A), and the Child and Adolescent Suicide Potential Index (CASPI).

Treatment of Aggression

Violent and out-of-control behavior is another common psychiatric emergency. Utilize the assessment above for determination of acute dangerousness. Treatment essentials are elaborated in Table 21.6.

TABLE 21.6. Treatment Essentials for Violent Youth

1. Determine cause of out-of-control and violent behavior. Ensure there is not an organic delirium or acute substance intoxication.
2. If the child is at acute risk of harm to self or others, safe and appropriate use of seclusion or restraint or medications (commonly an atypical antipsychotic with or without a benzodiazepine or diphenhydramine may be used).
3. Hospitalize if there is overt threat or aggression, especially with access to weapons, active psychosis, or inability to calm. Even if the aggressive behavior resolves in the emergency room, the risk for harming others in the home (e.g., a baby) and for a rapid re-escalation of aggressive behavior must be determined.
4. After safety is ensured, the goal of treatment is to address the underlying cause of out-of-control behavior. Use medication therapy, anger management training, parent-management training, and other interventions on a longer term basis.
5. If hospitalization is not immediately required, formulate a safe disposition plan, including rapid follow-up care and assessment of the need for child protective service involvement for acute issues in the family.
6. Ensure follow-up for regular treatment with a multimodal and multidisciplinary team.
7. Rating scales, such as the Overt Aggression Scale (OAS), may be helpful for ongoing monitoring of aggressive potential.

22 ▾ Child Neglect and Abuse

Essential Concepts
- All assessments of children and adolescents should include an evaluation for abuse or neglect.
- Children may be reluctant to disclose abuse. Information from multiple sources (including school, primary care physician, siblings, babysitter, child, parent, and protective services) may be indicated.
- Ask the child directly about means of discipline at home.
- Ask the child directly about having been touched in private places or asked to do things to other people's privates.

CLINICAL DESCRIPTION

Despite laws to protect them, the number of abused and neglected children in the United States has increased dramatically—likely due to an increase in maltreated children as well as increase in ascertainment and reporting. An estimated almost 900,000 reports of child maltreatment were substantiated in 2002. Of these, 60% involved child neglect, 20% physical abuse, 10% sexual abuse, and 7% emotional maltreatment (see Table 22.1). An estimated 1,400 children died of maltreatment in 2002. Eighty percent of perpetrators of physical abuse were parents, but less than 3% of all parent perpetrators were associated with sexual abuse. Girls are five times more likely to be the victim of sexual abuse. Infant boys have the highest rate of fatalities.

It is clear from these statistics that child abuse and neglect are of epidemic proportions. Developmental, psychiatric, and physical scars are the result. Chapter 19 reviews the psychiatric disorders associated with trauma. The present chapter will review risk and protective factors for child abuse and neglect, and discuss the role of individual assessment and intervention, as well as societal education and policy advocacy to help improve the care of infants, children, and adolescents in our country.

TABLE 22.1. Definition of Child Maltreatment: Child Abuse Prevention and Treatment Act

- *Physical abuse:* infliction of physical injury as the result of punching, beating, kicking, biting, burning, shaking, or otherwise intentionally harming a child
- *Sexual abuse:* fondling a child's genitals, intercourse, rape, sodomy, exhibitionism, and commercial exploitation through prostitution or the production of pornographic materials
- *Neglect:* failure to provide for a child's basic needs: 1) physical neglect, 2) educational neglect, 3) emotional neglect, and 4) medical neglect
- *Emotional abuse* (psychological/verbal abuse, mental injury): acts, failures to act, by parents or other caregivers that have caused or could cause serious behavioral, cognitive, emotional, or mental disorders

KEY POINT

Children often have a clear sense of needing to remain secretive about abuse or neglect. The child's fear of parents "getting in trouble," retribution for "telling," or the fear of being removed from the home all are incentives for a child to fail to disclose abuse.

TIP

Practice asking each child about abuse or neglect. The more you do it, the less uncomfortable you will feel, and the less anxious the child will be about answering. Suggestions include, "If you do something wrong, how do you get punished at home?" Also, "Has anyone ever hurt you?" Additionally, "Has anyone touched you in a way that made you feel scared? Has anyone touched your privates?" If you suspect that a child has been physically or sexually abused, you may have a small doll and ask, "Show me with this doll what happened to you." If it seems that legal charges may be pressed, you may want to curtail further investigation and refer to specialists who will do a forensic type of evaluation that may be used in court.

TABLE 22.2. Essentials of Assessment of Suspected
Abuse or Neglect

1. Physical examination for injuries that are not consistent with the
   history
   - Multiple injuries at various stages of healing
   - A history of failure to thrive
   - A history not consistent with the injury
   - Bruises in the pattern of a belt or fingers
   - Spiral fractures or rib fractures
   - Burns in a cigarette shape
   - Head and eye injuries, hemorrhages on fundoscopic
     examination
   - Unexplained serious abdominal injuries
   - Any injury to genitals
2. Full history from multiple informants (speak to them separately)
   regarding events, and assessment for inconsistency of reports
3. Assessment of new onset of sleep disturbance, startle reaction,
   regression, decline in academic and social functioning, or new
   psychiatric symptoms
4. Assessment for attachment issues, failure to thrive, PTSD,
   behavioral difficulties, sexual acting out or sexually provocative
   behaviors, or other psychiatric disorders

Assessment

Physicians should have a high index of suspicion for abuse
when evaluating an injured child whose presentation is atypical. The history may yield clues such as delayed seeking of
medical care, an explanation for an injury that does not fit the
injury or the child's developmental level, and frequently
changing stories (Table 22.2).

Etiology and Risk Factors

A multitude of factors place children at risk for maltreatment.
Current theories of child maltreatment integrate risk factors into
three primary systems: 1) the child; 2) the family; and 3) the
community and society. Although no child deserves to be mis-
treated, a child's characteristics may significantly elevate the likelihood of maltreatment. It is the complex interaction between
the child's risk factors and that of the family and society that lead
to maltreatment. Risk factors and protective factors are specified
in Tables 22.3 and 22.4.

TABLE 22.3. **Essential Risk Factors for Child Maltreatment**

1. Child factors
   - Premature birth and low birth weight, in utero exposures, birth anomalies
   - Difficult temperament
   - Physical/cognitive/emotional disability or chronic illness
   - ADHD, aggression, and behavior problems
   - Childhood trauma
   - Younger age
2. Family factors
   - Domestic violence
   - Poor family communication and problem-solving skills
   - Parent having been maltreated as a child
   - Highly stressed family—financial stress, single parent, lots of children in the home, low employability, disability
   - Parental psychopathology, substance abuse, poor impulse control
   - Inaccurate knowledge and expectations about child development
3. Social and environmental factors
   - Low socioeconomic status (SES), homelessness
   - Dangerous neighborhood
   - Social isolation and lack of support
   - Lack of access to health care and child care
   - Poor schools
   - Exposure to environmental toxins

 TIP

All mental health professionals, physicians, and teachers are mandated reporters. That means that you are legally required to report to the state protective service agency any suspected cases of child abuse or neglect.

 TIP

At times, children and adolescents will falsely accuse parents or others of abuse. Often the motivation (anger and revenge, or being triangulated between two families) may be obvious.

Mandated reporting to the state protective service agency is required if there is legitimate suspicion of abuse and neglect. The accusations may then be investigated to ascertain the credibility.

Treatment

The initial goal of treatment is to ensure that the child is safe and to prevent further abuse. This is typically done in concert with the protective service agencies. The child may be removed from the home and placed in foster care, a group home, or another out of the home living situation. The abuser will require treatment, close monitoring, and support if the child is to remain in the home or return to the home.

TABLE 22.4. Protective Factors to Prevent Child Maltreatment

1. Child factors
   - Ability to recognize danger and adapt
   - Ability to distance oneself from intense feelings
   - Ability to imagine oneself at a time and place in the future in which the perpetrator is no longer present
   - Good health
   - Average or above intelligence
   - Hobbies or interests
   - Good peer relationships and social skills
   - Easy temperament
   - Positive self-esteem
   - Internal locus of control
2. Family factors
   - Secure attachment
   - Parental working through of their own abuse histories
   - Supportive family environment
   - Household rules and supervision
   - Extended family support
   - High parental education
   - Family expectation of prosocial behavior
3. Social and environmental factors
   - Middle to high SES
   - Access to health care and child care
   - Sufficient housing

(Continued)

TABLE 22.4. **Protective Factors to Prevent Child Maltreatment** (*continued*)

- Steady parental employment
- Good schools
- Religious affiliation
- Adults outside the family who serve as positive role models/mentors

---

Therapies for maltreated children are individualized, based on diagnoses generated from a complete developmental psychiatric or multidisciplinary evaluation that incorporates a developmental psychiatric component. Medication therapy may be appropriate to treat the secondary target symptoms, such as anxiety, depression, or agitation. Early detection and intervention improves prognosis. Children may remain in the home safely if the parents are highly motivated to receive help via intensive in-home supports and are receiving their own psychiatric or substance abuse treatment, and the abuse was not life-threatening or severe.

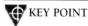 KEY POINT

Physicians must provide the advocacy required to ensure that risk factors for child abuse and neglect are minimized. Ensuring access to care, providing supports to families with young children, parenting classes, appropriate and safe housing, and quality day-care are protective factors that minimize the potential for serious abuse and neglect. The scars of abuse and neglect can be avoided in many instances. Parents generally love and care for their children, and abuse them only when their own stress is overwhelming. Advocacy by physicians, mental health professionals, teachers, and families is needed to provide the social and community supports that will help families function in a more nurturing manner toward children.

TREATMENT

23 ▼ Principles of Treatment Planning

Essential Concepts

- An appropriate treatment plan emanates from a thorough psychiatric evaluation.
- Sensitive feedback about the results of the evaluation sets the stage for providing treatment recommendations.
- A therapeutic alliance must be forged with both the patient and his or her parents or guardians.
- Setting a stage of mutual respect and open communication at the outset of treatment begins an alliance that may be the most powerful therapeutic tool you have.

CLINICAL DESCRIPTION

When parents or guardians bring their child for evaluation by a mental health professional (especially a physician) they may be riddled with guilt, fearful of the diagnosis, and anxious about the potential of being blamed for the child's difficulties. They may see their child's failings as evidence of their inadequacy as parents.

The reason and source of referral for a child or adolescent receiving a psychiatric evaluation is essential to determine. Ask why the family is coming now. Begin the evaluation with as much clarity as possible about the process—first the evaluation, and then the feedback and recommendations for treatment. Treatment of psychiatric disorders tends to be shrouded in mystery and ambiguity for many people. Parents may fear the use of medication. They may be concerned about stigma. Clarify these issues early and often.

The feedback about evaluation findings should begin a dialogue about the child's strengths, weaknesses, diagnosis, and target symptoms.

KEY POINT

Clarify the nature of confidentiality of treatment with the child and the family. In general, the younger the child the more that is shared about the general progress of treatment. It is important that the parents have a clear understanding of the treatment goals and methods, such that they understand the process of psychotherapy and pharmacotherapy. There can be confidentiality as to the content of the therapy unless there is a potential that the child is self-destructive or destructive to others. Suicidality, antisocial behaviors, sexual promiscuity, and substance use are issues that do not have confidentiality if the child is at serious risk of harm. Usually it is reassuring to the child and promotes a sense of safety when the limits of confidentiality are elaborated.

 TIP

In general, the postevaluation feedback is with parents and guardians first. However, with adolescents, it is advised that they have the option of being present at meetings with the parents when the findings of the evaluation and recommendations are being made. It is also helpful to discuss with an adolescent what they would like their parents to be told about the content of your meetings with him or her, and to give some feedback about the issues you think he or she is dealing with. The general approach is to join with the adolescent in working together for common goals.

 KEY POINT

The intensity of the treatment (inpatient, partial hospital, in-home services, or outpatient therapy) is the first determination. Secondly, determine whether treatment will be sequential (for example, starting with psychotherapy and only adding medication if the therapy does not work), or multimodal (starting several interventions at once). Much depends on the acuity and functional impairment of the symptoms. Many children require multimodal treatment in a variety of systems (family, individual, school, etc.). The physician should help coordinate the treatment and be an active member of the treatment team.

TABLE 23.1. Setting the Stage for Treatment

- Set aside sufficient time to discuss the results of your evaluation of the child. A therapeutic alliance with the parents may be initiated via open communication and a nonblaming, but clear diagnostic formulation of the components of their child's strengths as well as challenges.
- Formulate a treatment plan with goals and objectives. Use a biopsychosocial formulation to focus your treatment plan.
  - Biological—what is the psychiatric diagnosis? Identify if there is a biological treatment (medication) that may be helpful. Is there need for further testing (psychological, laboratory, etc.) to assess physical health and biological strengths and vulnerabilities?
  - Psychological—what are the psychological symptoms? Are there psychotherapeutic techniques that will be helpful?
  - Family and social issues may be a primary target of treatment. Family conflict is often an issue. Friends, social network, and school may be other areas of need.
- Set priorities—choose to target the most impairing symptoms first.
  - Safety of the child, including risk of harm to self or others.
  - Symptoms that are likely to worsen without rapid treatment (such as school avoidance).
  - Problems that are most urgent to the child and family.
  - Symptoms that are most amenable to treatment.
- Parents, and usually the child, should help determine which treatment strategy to follow. Parental motivation or ability to carry out a treatment plan is a primary factor.
- The treatment plan should be consistent with the family's resources (time, money, and emotional).
- Discuss the evidence base for treatment. If there are treatments that have been demonstrated to be effective, discuss them with the parents. Risks of the intervention as well as benefits (and risks of no intervention) should be discussed. If there isn't much evidence for a treatment, say so. Also say why you are recommending the treatment(s) you are.
- Treatment planning (and communication about treatment progress) is an ongoing process. Continue to reassess the child and his or her response to interventions and make appropriate modifications.

Psychopharmacology

> **Essential Concepts**
> - Medication may be an important component of a multimodal treatment plan for a child suffering from behavioral and emotional problems.
> - For all psychotropics used, there should be a careful consideration of risks and benefits of the treatment with the family/guardian and education and assent of the child.
> - Rating forms of symptoms prior to and following the initiation of medication may be helpful in quantifying effectiveness as well as side effects.
> - Take a careful medical and medication/substance history prior to the initiation of any medication, with laboratory, ECG, or other tests as appropriate.

It is part of the cure to wish to be cured.

—Lucius Annaeus Seneca

GENERAL PRINCIPLES AND CLINICAL CONSIDERATIONS

The essential consideration in using medications for the treatment of psychiatric disorders in children and adolescents is being clear what the diagnosis and target symptoms are, knowing the risks and benefits, and being thoughtful and careful about medication use. While this is important for all of medicine, it is even truer in the treatment of children, whose bodies and nervous systems are not yet fully developed.

Pharmacotherapy should be part of a broader treatment plan in which consideration is given to all aspects of the child's life. It should not replace psychosocial and educational interventions. Likewise, medication should not be thought of as the treatment of last resort, when everything else has failed. Realistic expectations of pharmacotherapy based on a clear definition of which target symptoms may be effectively ameliorated as well as what cannot be reasonably expected (e.g., changing the child's attitude) are the ingredients for successful intervention.

Even as there needs to be care taken in using medication, we also know that untreated disorders (such as depression, mania, and psychosis) have worse prognoses. There is evidence that early detection and medication intervention with prodromal schizophrenia may improve lifetime prognosis and functioning. We also know that children who are unable to pay attention will miss out academically and socially on early developmental tasks. Thus, risks of using medication must be weighed against not only the benefits but also the risk of not treating, which may be chronicity and social incapacitation.

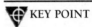 **KEY POINT**

Many of the medications used for the treatment of psychiatric disorders in children and adolescents are considered "off-label," or not approved by the U.S. Food and Drug Administration (FDA) for the pediatric population. For many medications, the intensive testing required for FDA approval has not been sought by the medication manufacturers. For this reason, medications determined to be effective with adults are used with children. Because children are not just "miniature adults," the medications should be used more judiciously, carefully, and only with clear indications and target symptoms.

Evaluation and Treatment

The sine qua non of all psychiatric care is a thorough evaluation, using multiple informants. This includes ensuring good physical health, and getting baseline laboratory and physical assessment data, as indicated. Table 24.1 highlights the essentials of evaluation prior to the use of pharmacotherapy.

Once the decision has been made that pharmacotherapy is appropriate for the symptoms and functional disability with which the child or adolescent presents, follow the plan for pharmacotherapy outlined in Table 24.2.

TABLE 24.1. Evaluation Essentials for the Use of Pharmacotherapy

1. Conduct a comprehensive psychiatric evaluation of the child or adolescent, including information from multiple sources, assessment of the family, and family history of psychiatric and medical disorders.
2. Provide careful diagnostic and psychiatric symptom review with the patient and caregivers.
3. Ensure a physical examination.
4. Collect baseline laboratory and physical assessment data where warranted. Consider baseline rating scales of target symptoms.
5. Determine indicated nonpharmacologic interventions for the diagnosed disorder.
6. Consider the risks and benefits of pharmacotherapy.
7. Consider the risks and benefits of specific medications relevant to the disorder.
8. Conduct a formal consent procedure with the parent and youth. Give handouts on medications, where appropriate.

TABLE 24.2. Essentials of Pharmacotherapy

1. Review the patient's (and pertinent family) medical history, drug allergies, and past drug reactions.
2. Identify treatable symptoms and establish treatment goals.
3. Initiate medications at low doses and assess dosing schedule (for ease, effectiveness, and to minimize side effects).
4. Monitor therapy regularly.
   - Ask patient and parents about presence of adverse reactions and side effects.
   - Perform routine physical assessments (blood pressure, height, weight, etc.).
   - Use rating scales to assess side effects, as available.
5. Limit and manage side effects.
   - Start medications at low doses and titrate slowly.
   - Avoid adding medications that may cause drug interactions.
   - Identify need for medications that treat side effects (e.g., benztropine, diphenhydramine).
6. Determine treatment duration.
   - Evaluate effectiveness of medication and dosage after 2–6 weeks.
   - Duration of therapy—reevaluate need for medication every 6 months.

(Continued)

TABLE 24.2. **Essentials of Pharmacotherapy** (*continued*)

7. Minimize duplicate therapy and polypharmacy.
   * Monotherapy is preferred when possible.
   * Consider potential drug–drug interactions when combining medications.
8. Coordinate care with the patient, caretakers, all health care and mental health care providers, and the family pharmacist.

MAJOR CLASSES OF MEDICATIONS USED IN CHILD AND ADOLESCENT PSYCHIATRY

Stimulant Medications

The stimulant medications act to enhance dopamine and noradrenergic transmission. They improve both cognitive and behavioral functioning. They are considered the first-line medications in the treatment of attention deficit hyperactivity disorder (ADHD). Stimulants are the most prescribed psychotropic agents for children in the United States.

The stimulant medications come in short and longer acting preparations. The most commonly reported side effects of stimulant medications are appetite suppression and sleep disturbance. Less frequently, mood disturbance, headaches, abdominal discomfort, increased lethargy, and fatigue or "spaciness" have been reported. There may be increases in heart rate and blood pressure, and monitoring is suggested. Additionally, all stimulants may exacerbate tics. Although the etiology remains unclear, some ADHD children taking stimulants may demonstrate growth delay. "Drug holidays" (summers or other periods of time not taking the stimulant) typically remediate that delay. Table 24.3 gives information relevant to the use of stimulant medication in clinical practice.

 TIP

There has been concern raised in Canada and later in the United States that Adderal XR and possibly other stimulants may increase the risk of sudden death. Although epidemiologically this has not been substantiated, a careful individual and family history of heart arrhythmias and monitoring of heart rate, blood pressure, and EKG, as indicated, are advised for Adderal XR and the other stimulant medications.

TABLE 24.3. Stimulant Medications

Drug	Chemical Effect	Average Daily Dose Range	Pharmacokinetic Parameters (duration)	Monitoring
Amphetamine Mixtures				
Adderall	Blocks reuptake of DA and NE, inhibits MAO	2.5–40 mg 1–3 divided doses	4–6 h	Blood pressure, height, weight
Adderall XR		10–30 mg QAM	12 h	
Dextroamphetamine				
Dexedrine	Blocks reuptake of DA and NE, inhibits MAO	5–40 mg 1–3 divided doses	4–6 h	Blood pressure, height, weight
Dexedrine spansules		5–40 mg QD	6–8 h	
Methylphenidate				
Concerta	Blocks reuptake of DA	18–54 mg QAM	12 h	Blood pressure, height, weight
Metadate CD		20–60 mg QAM	9 h	

(Continued)

187

TABLE 24.3. Stimulant Medications (*continued*)

Drug	Chemical Effect	Average Daily Dose Range	Pharmacokinetic Parameters (duration)	Monitoring
Amphetamine Mixtures				
Focalin		5–20 mg 2 divided doses	3–5 h	Blood pressure, height, weight
Ritalin IR		5–60 mg 2–3 divided doses	3–5 h	
Ritalin SR		20 mg QD	8 h	
Other				
Cylert (pemoline)	Blocks reuptake of DA	37.5–112.5 mg QD	6–8 h	Liver enzymes, height, weight

DA, dopamine; NE, norepinephrine; MAO, monoamine oxidase.

188

Antidepressant Medications

Antidepressant therapy is composed of four main drug classes: tricyclic antidepressants (TCAs), selective serotonin reuptake inhibitors (SSRIs), newer atypical antidepressants, and monoamine oxidase inhibitors (MAOIs). The MAOIs are associated with a number of dietary and therapeutic restrictions that make the use of this medication in children and adolescents unpopular. This section will focus on the other three categories of antidepressants.

In clinical practice, antidepressants are essential options for patients with unipolar depression or anxiety. Care must be taken to assess for a previous history of mania-like symptoms and to monitor for activation and fluctuations in suicidality with treatment. The SSRIs have been demonstrated effective in the treatment of depression. The other classes of medication may be beneficial for an individual patient, but have less evidence of effectiveness for depression. However, the TCAs and atypical antidepressant medications may be useful for treatment of other psychiatric disorders, such as anxiety, enuresis, insomnia, and ADHD. Each antidepressant class has a unique mechanism of action and side-effect profile. Information regarding the use of antidepressants with young people is summarized in Table 24.4.

 TIP

Remember that antidepressant effectiveness is not immediately apparent. Initial improvement can be expected after 4 to 6 weeks of pharmacotherapy, but substantial improvement may not be apparent until up to 12 weeks. Once the patient has achieved a remission of symptoms, the antidepressant should be continued for a duration of at least 9 months in order to prevent relapse. Patients with three or more episodes of depression and those whose first episode was unusually severe are at high risk of recurrence and should be considered for maintenance therapy. Watch carefully for "switching" or induction of mania.

🔑 KEY POINT

Among the antidepressants, only fluoxetine is approved by the FDA for use in treating major depressive disorder in pediatric patients. Fluoxetine, sertraline, fluvoxamine, and clomipramine are approved for OCD in pediatric patients. Antidepressant

TABLE 24.4. Antidepressant Medications

Drug	Chemical Effect	Average Daily Dose Range	Side Effects	Monitoring
Tricyclic Antidepressants (TCAs)				
Amitriptyline (Elavil) (tertiary TCA)	5HT, ±NE	Children: 1–3 mg/kg/day in three divided doses Adolescents: 25–100 mg/day	Anticholinergic side effects, orthostatic hypotension, sedation,	EKG, CBC, blood pressure, heart rate, weight, plasma concentrations
Imipramine (Tofranil) (tertiary TCA)		Children: 1.5–5 mg/kg/day in 1 to 4 divided doses Adolescents: 25 to 100 mg/day	GI intolerance, weight gain, sexual dysfunction	
Nortriptyline (Pamelor) (secondary TCA)	NE, ±5HT	Children: 1–3 mg/kg/day in 3–4 divided doses Adolescents: 30–150 mg/day in 3–4 divided doses	Same as above; less anticholinergic and sedative effects	
Selective Serotonin Reuptake Inhibitors (SSRIs)				
Citalopram (Celexa)	5HT	No dosing information available for children	GI intolerance, sexual dysfunction, activation, mania, sleep disturbance	Weight, liver function, drug interactions, manic symptoms, suicidality
Escitalopram (Lexapro)	5HT	(5–40 mg/day is usual)		
Fluoxetine (Prozac)	5HT	5–40 mg/day (can be given three times a week)		

Fluvoxamine (Luvox)	5HT	50–200 mg/day (may need multiple daily dosing)	GI intolerance, sexual dysfunction, activation, mania, sleep disturbance	Weight, liver function, drug interactions, manic symptoms, suicidality
Paroxetine (Paxil)	5HT	5–20 mg/day (limited data)		
Sertraline (Zoloft)	5HT	Children: 25–100 mg/day Adolescents: 50–100 mg/day		
Atypical Antidepressants				
Bupropion (Wellbutrin, Wellbutrin SR, Wellbutrin XL)	NE, DA	Limited data with IR product in pediatric patients; typical adult dose is 100 mg TID	Agitation, insomnia, GI intolerance	Weight, blood pressure, seizure threshold (Contraindicated with bulimia)
Venlafaxine (Effexor, Effexor XR)	5HT, NE	No dosing information available for children	GI intolerance, sexual dysfunction, activation, mania, sleep disturbance, hypertension	Weight, blood pressure, drug interactions
Mirtazapine (Remeron)	5HT, NE	No dosing information available for children	Somnolence, weight gain	Lipids, weight, agranulocytosis
Nefazodone (Serzone)	5HT	No dosing information available for children	GI intolerance, insomnia, agitation	Liver function, drug interactions

5HT, serotonin; NE, norepinephrine; DA, dopamine; EKG, electrocardiogram; CBC, complete blood count; IR, immediate release.

medication may effectively ameliorate depression in youth. In the Treatment for Adolescents with Depression (TADS) study, 71% improved with both fluoxetine and CBT, 60% improved with fluoxetine alone, 43% improved with CBT alone, and 34% improved with placebo.

◈ KEY POINT

In October 2004, the U.S. Food and Drug Administration (FDA) issued a black box warning for all antidepressants used in the pediatric "age range." This was prompted by concerns that antidepressant use may exacerbate suicidal thinking and behaviors in vulnerable children and adolescents who are treated with these medications. The FDA warning emphasizes the need for careful clinical monitoring of young patients receiving antidepressants. FDA recommended guidelines include weekly monitoring for the first 4 weeks after initiating antidepressant medication, then every other week for the second 4 weeks, then assessed every 3 months while on the medication. Assess for worsening of depression or suicidality and symptoms of activation (anxiety, agitation, disinhibition, panic, irritability, insomnia, akathisia, or mania/hypomania). Of note, there were no completed suicides by antidepressant users in the studies cited by the FDA.

Mood Stabilizers

There are three commonly used and well-studied mood stabilizers: lithium, valproate, and carbamazepine. Of the three, only lithium is FDA approved for the treatment of bipolar disorder in adolescents (over the age of 12). Valproate is becoming increasingly popular for the treatment of mania in children and adolescents. It appears to be as effective and may be better tolerated in some patients. Information regarding the clinical use of these three major mood stabilizers is summarized in Table 24.5.

Anti-Anxiety Medications

Drugs with anxiolytic activity include benzodiazepines, buspirone, TCAs, SSRIs, alpha-2a agonists, such as clonidine or guanfacine, and beta-blockers. Of these, only benzodiazepines and buspirone are specifically considered anxiolytics.

TABLE 24.5. Mood Stabilizer Medications

Drug	Chemical Effect	Average Daily Dose Range	Side Effects	Monitoring
Lithium carbonate (Lithobid, Eskalith)	5HT, ±NE	Children: 15–60 mg/kg/day in 3–4 divided doses. Adolescents: 600–1800 mg/day in 3–4 divided doses or 2 divided doses for sustained-release products	Sedation, thirst, polyuria, polydipsia, weight gain, GI intolerance, tremor, hypothyroidism, seizures, acne	EKG, CBC, electrolytes, renal function tests, thyroid function tests, weight, plasma concentrations **Serum levels:** Acute mania: 0.8–1.5 mEq/L Maintenance: 0.6–1 mEq/L
Valproate, valproic acid (Depakote, Depakene)	GABA	30–60 mg/kg/day in 2–3 divided doses.	Sedation, thrombocytopenia, alopecia, nausea, weight gain, tremor, GI upset, hepatotoxicity, agranulocytosis, neutropenia	CBC with platelets, liver function tests, weight, menses, plasma concentrations **Serum level:** 50–125 µg/mL
Carbamazepine (Tegretol, Carbatrol)	Multiple CNS effects	Children: 10–20 mg/kg/day in 3–4 divided doses. Adolescents: 400–800 mg/day in 2–3 divided doses	Dizziness, rash, impaired coordination, slurred speech, ataxia, drowsiness, nausea, vomiting, agranulocytosis, hepatotoxicity	CBC with platelets, EKG, weight, plasma concentrations **Serum level:** 8–12 µg/mL

5HT, serotonin; NE, norepinephrine; GABA, γ aminobutyric acid; EKG, electrocardiogram; CBC, complete blood count.

Benzodiazepines are used in the treatment of acute anxiety, panic, and sleep disorders, and may be useful for acute treatment of neuroleptic-induced akathisia. Benzodiazepines potentiate the inhibitory effects of GABA. The disadvantages of benzodiazepines are their sedation, disinhibition, and psychological and physical dependence. For these reasons, benzodiazepines are rarely used in child and adolescent psychiatry as maintenance medications, but may have utility in the acute management of severe anxiety (such as debilitating school-related anxiety) for a brief period of time.

Buspirone is an azapirone anxiolytic. Unlike benzodiazepines, the anxiolytic effect of buspirone is not immediate and can take up to 2 to 3 weeks. Advantages are that it is not associated with dependence or withdrawal reactions and has no demonstrated potential for abuse. However, clinically buspirone may not be as effective as an anxiolytic, and data regarding its use in children are sparse. Information about the use of anxiolytics in clinical practice is summarized in Table 24.6.

Antipsychotic Medications

Antipsychotic medications are used to treat children with serious psychopathology including psychotic disorders, depression with psychotic features, mania, autism spectrum disorders, Tourette disorder, self-injurious behaviors, and severe aggressive behaviors.

There are two general classes of antipsychotics used in clinical practice: the traditional antipsychotics and the atypical antipsychotics. Both categories of antipsychotics effectively treat the hallmarks of psychosis, that is, the positive or active symptoms including hallucinations, delusions, bizarre behavior, disordered thinking, and severe agitation. The newer atypical antipsychotics are more successful at ameliorating the negative symptoms of schizophrenia such as apathy and avolition. It is this latter action plus their less severe side effect profile that has led to the atypical antipsychotics replacing the traditional antipsychotics as first-line antipsychotic medications.

Potential long-term complications of most atypical antipsychotics include hyperprolactinemia, extrapyramidal symptoms (EPS), and tardive dyskinesia (TD), although TD is less common with atypical antipsychotics than with the typicals. Additionally, the FDA has issued a warning that all of the atypical antipsychotics carry a risk of precipitating type-2 diabetes. Olanzapine and clozapine are associated with the greatest weight gain and glucose intolerance. Ziprasidone has

TABLE 24.6. Antianxiety Medications

Drug	Chemical Effect	Average Daily Dose Range	Side Effects	Monitoring
Benzodiazepines				
Alprazolam (Xanax)	GABA	0.375–3 mg/day in 3 divided doses	Sedation, disinhibition, drowsiness, incoordination, confusion, memory impairment	HR, RR, BP, CBC, liver function
Clonazepam (Klonopin)	GABA	0.1–0.2 mg/kg/day in 2 divided doses		
Diazepam (Valium)	GABA	0.12–0.8 mg/kg/day in 3 divided doses		
Lorazepam (Ativan)	GABA	0.02–0.1 mg/kg every 4–8 h		
Nonbenzodiazepines				
Buspirone (BuSpar)	5HT	0.3–0.6 mg/kg/day in 2 divided doses	Dizziness, headache, lightheadedness, nausea	Liver function, renal function

GABA, γ-aminobutyric acid; 5HT, serotonin; HR, heart rate; RR, respiratory rate; BP, blood pressure; CBC, complete blood count.

the fewest metabolic side effects, but must be monitored for prolonged conduction (QTc) on electrocardiogram. Aripiprazol reportedly causes the least hyperphagia and therefore should have a decreased risk of metabolic syndrome.

For the use of all antipsychotics, monitoring with the Abnormal Involuntary Movement Scale (AIMS) for the development of tardive dyskinesia and the Simpson-Angus Scale (SAS) for extrapyramidal symptoms is recommended. These are found in Appendix 1.

Information regarding the use of antipsychotics in clinical practice is summarized in Table 24.7.

Other Agents

A variety of other agents have been used in the treatment of child and adolescent psychiatric disorders. A few of these agents will be briefly discussed and are summarized in Table 24.8.

Atomoxetine (Strattera) is the first nonstimulant medication approved for the treatment of ADHD. Although its true mechanism of action is unknown, it is thought to be related to the selective inhibition of the presynaptic norepinephrine transporter. Although it has not demonstrated superior effectiveness to stimulant medications, it may be useful for youth who do not tolerate stimulant medication well, or who suffer from both ADHD and tics.

The alpha-adrenergic agonists, clonidine and guanfacine, were originally used as blood pressure medications, but have been used widely in child and adolescent psychiatry. They are the first-line treatment for tics. These medications may also have utility for treating the hyperactivity and impulsivity of ADHD. Additionally, the adrenergic agonist medications have been used successfully in treating some anxiety disorders, such as posttraumatic stress disorder, in which there is physiological arousal with increased sympathetic outflow. Clonidine is especially helpful in settling youth at night so they can sleep. Other uses have included the control of aggression toward self and others in youth with developmental disorders.

Diphenhydramine (Benadryl) and hydroxyzine (Atarax, Vistaril) are antihistamines used for a variety of psychiatric disorders and side effects of psychiatric medications. Diphenhydramine has been used effectively to treat sleep disturbances, anxiety, and EPS. Hydroxyzine is commonly used for the treatment of anxiety. Both medications may be activating or may cause visual perceptual disturbance in a small group of children who are sensitive to the central anticholinergic effect.

TABLE 24.7. Antipsychotic Medications

Drug	Chemical Effect	Average Daily Dose Range	Side Effects	Monitoring
Traditional Antipsychotics—Lower Potency Agent				
Chlorpromazine (Thorazine)	DA	0.5–1 mg/kg every 4–6 hours	Anticholinergic effects, orthostasis, sedation, EPS, NMS	CBC, BP, AIMS, SAS, EKG
Traditional Antipsychotics—Higher Potency Agent				
Haloperidol (Haldol)	DA	0.01–0.15 mg/kg/day in 2–3 divided doses	EPS, NMS hyperprolactinemia	EKG, BP, CBC, electrolytes, AIMS, SAS
Atypical Antipsychotics				
Aripiprazole (Abilify)	DA	No data in children; adult dose: 10–15 mg/day	Headache, akathisia, sleep disturbance, orthostasis	Weight, BMI, glucose, fasting lipids, BP, AIMS, SAS, EKG
Risperidone (Risperdal)	5HT, DA	Adult dose: 2–6 mg/day	Orthostasis, hyperprolactinemia, weight gain, EPS, hyperlipidemia	
Olanzapine (Zyprexa)	5HT, DA	Adult dose: 10–20 mg/day	Sedation, weight gain, hyperglycemia, hyperlipidemia	

(Continued)

197

TABLE 24.7. Antipsychotic Medications (*continued*)

Drug	Chemical Effect	Average Daily Dose Range	Side Effects	Monitoring
Quetiapine (Seroquel)	5HT, DA	Adult dose: 150–800 mg/day	Sedation, orthostasis, weight gain	Weight, BMI, glucose, fasting lipids, BP, AIMS, SAS
Ziprasidone (Geodon)	5HT, DA	Adult dose: 80–160 mg/day	Sedation, akathisia	
Clozapine (Clozaril)	5HT, DA	Adult dose: 200–900 mg/day	Orthostasis, weight gain, hyperglycemia, hyperlipidemia	

DA, dopamine; 5HT, serotonin; EPS, extrapyramidal symptoms; NMS, neuroleptic malignant syndrome; CBC, complete blood count; BP, blood pressure; EKG, electrocardiogram; BMI, Body Mass Index; AIMS, Abnormal Involuntary Movement Scale; SAS, Simpson Angus Scale.

TABLE 24.8. Other Medications

Drug	Chemical Effect	Average Daily Dose Range	Side Effects	Monitoring
Clonidine (Catapres)	Presynaptic alpha adrenergic agonist	3–10 µg/kg in 2–4 div doses	Sedation, hypotension, headache, dizziness, dry mouth Irritability, nausea, depression, bradycardia, skin irritation with patch, rebound HTN	BP, pulse, weight, EKG if history of CV disease in child or family
Guanfacine (Tenex)	Presynaptic alpha adrenergic agonist	15–90 µg/kg 1–2 div doses	Same as Clonidine, but less hypotension and sedation	BP, pulse, weight, EKG if history of CV disease in child or family
Atomoxetine (Strattera)	NorE reuptake inhibitor	0.5–1.8 mg/kg 1–2 div doses	GI discomfort, decreased appetite, rhinitis, headache, lethargy, mild insomnia	BP, pulse, weight
Diphenhydramine (Benadryl)	H1 antagonist	25–300 mg/day 1–4 div doses	Sedation, dizziness, dry mouth, constipation, blurred vision, lowered seizure threshold with very high doses	No specific tests
Hydroxyzine (Atarax, Vistaril)	H1 antagonist	10–100 mg/day 1–4 div doses	Same as diphenhydramine	No specific tests

Psychosocial Interventions

Essential Concepts
- Psychosocial interventions include the full range of nonpharmacologic treatments that engage the child, adolescent, and family in the process of adaptive change.
- The type of psychosocial intervention recommended depends on the presenting symptoms and evidence for the type of intervention that works best for the child's specific difficulty.
- Use goals and objectives for treatment to remain focused and to ensure ongoing assessment of effectiveness or needed modifications.
- In working with children and adolescents, both the parents or guardians and the identified patient need to be engaged in the therapeutic process.

Whenever two people meet there are really six people present. There is each man as he sees himself, each man as the other person sees him, and each man as he really is.

—William James

GENERAL PRINCIPLES AND CLINICAL CONSIDERATIONS

Psychotherapeutic interventions are indicated for the majority of psychiatric disorders in children and adolescents. For psychotherapy to be effective with youth, the parents or guardians need to be engaged—to be educated about their child's problems and share a vision with the therapist regarding the goals of treatment and the therapeutic interventions. In fact, family therapy or working with the parents to help them learn and utilize more effective parenting skills may be the modality of choice for some difficulties.

A key to effective psychosocial treatment is to choose the types of intervention that are most helpful for the problem at hand. This requires familiarity with the range of levels of care, as well as a wide variety of therapeutic techniques and their indications.

Practical Aspects of Psychotherapeutic Applications

Ideally, the mental health service delivery system provides an integrated continuum of care at a variety of levels of intensity and utilizing individualized modalities specific to the child's particular needs. The child and family can easily access appropriate services as the clinical situation warrants.

Although the ideal continuum of services may not be available, children live in systems (family, school, etc.), and it is incumbent upon the child and adolescent psychiatrist to assess and help the child and family access needed services. Child and adolescent psychiatric disorders cannot be successfully treated unless the family dynamics and the system environment are considered. Often, the therapist coordinates with the school, child, family, social service agency, pediatrician, juvenile court personnel and/or any other significant providers in the child's life.

Choosing appropriate modalities of treatment is informed by a thorough psychiatric evaluation. An appreciation of the child's level of physical, cognitive, and emotional development is required to set appropriate goals and tailor effective interventions. All therapeutic interventions focus on helping the child and family gain skills required for more adaptive and healthy development and coping, and enhancing his or her overall level of functioning. Table 25.1 summarizes the types of psychosocial treatments that are indicated for various types of difficulties.

Individual Psychotherapies

While there are many forms of psychotherapy, all of them follow a basic psychotherapeutic process, which has been well described in a 1982 publication by the Group for the Advancement of Psychiatry Committee on Child Psychiatry. Table 25.2 outlines this five-stage process.

The Psychotherapeutic Process

Establishing a working relationship, or engagement period, is the first stage of any psychotherapy. This process begins with the very first encounter. In transference, your patient unconsciously

TABLE 25.1. Essentials of Psychosocial Treatments for Children and Adolescents

Type of Treatment Used	Indications	Modalities Used
Hospitalization	Acute safety issues (to self or others) Functionally incapacitating psychiatric symptoms Lack of stabilization in less intensive treatment	Pharmacotherapy Individual psychotherapy Milieu therapy/behavioral therapy Group therapy Family therapy Education assessment or maintneance
Residential treatment	Chronic and severe behavioral and emotional problems that cannot be adequately addressed in outpatient setting	Same
Partial hospitalization or day treatment	Patient is safe to live at home, foster home, or group home but requires intensive therapeutic supports	May or may not include a school program Pharmacotherapy Individual psychotherapy Family involvement Group therapy
In-home behavioral treatment	Patient is safe to live at home, but entire family requires intensive supports to maintain home safety and foster the child's appropriate and healthy development	In-home behavioral plans Psychoeducation about parenting, child development In-home therapy of child and family Pharmacotherapy as appropriate

Wrap-around services	Child with complex mental health and psychosocial needs	In-home services are component
	To avoid need for institutional care	Integration with social services to ensure entitlements and housing
		Crisis intervention teams
		Respite services
		Coordinated community services
Psychotherapy		
Individual therapy	Youth who has difficulty forming positive relationships with adults or who is in crisis	Supportive therapy
	Verbal youngsters who are struggling to deal with recurrent maladaptive relationship issues or traumatic events	Psychodynamically oriented therapy
	Verbal youngsters who are working through relationship and personality development issues	Psychoanalysis
	Circumscribed problems of recent onset	Time-limited therapy
	Depressed, anxious, or conduct-disordered youth	CBT, ITP, and other EBPs
	Behavior or developmentally disordered youth	Behavior therapy
Group therapy	Single stressor, single psychiatric disorder, or focus of difficulty	Social and coping skills groups
		Problem solving and anger management
		Mutual support and insights

(Continued)

TABLE 25.1. Essentials of Psychosocial Treatments for Children and Adolescents (*continued*)

Type of Treatment Used	Indications	Modalities Used
Family therapy	Family with poor communication and structure	Structural family therapy
	Resistant families with rigid coping and relating	Strategic family therapy
	Family that does not understand the nature of the child's difficulties and how to be helpful	Psychoeducational family therapy
	Family with child who has learned negative behaviors	Behavior therapy
	Parents who do not have skills in behavior management of their children	Parent Management Training (PMT)

CBT, cognitive behavioral therapy (there is trauma-focused CBT, as well as specific CBT techniques for depression, anxiety disorders, and obsessive-compulsive disorder); ITP, interpersonal therapy; EBPs, evidence-based psychotherapies.

TABLE 25.2. The Stages of the Psychotherapeutic Process

Stage of Psychotherapy	Tasks of the Stage
Establishing the working relationship	• Engaging with the child and parents • Identifying any transference or countertransference problems • Developing trust in treatment relationship
Analysis of the problem and its cause	• Examination of the child's life • Assist the patient in developing a problem list • Assist the parents in developing a problem list • Integrate the problem list for next stage
Developing an explanation of the problem	• Describe the possible reasons for the identified problems • Outline the work needed to be done • Define the rules for the working relationship (appointment times, billing, cancellations, etc.) • Agree on a treatment plan

(Continued)

TABLE 25.2. The Stages of the Psychotherapeutic Process (continued)

Stage of Psychotherapy	Tasks of the Stage
Establishing and implementing the formula for change and selected formula for change	• Implement the treatment plan (prescription for change) • Readjust formula for change as indicated • If there is now progress, review and adjust initial problem list
Termination	• Review the reasons for entering treatment • Summarize what was helpful and not helpful in solving presenting problems • Consolidate therapeutic gains with praise • Address any loss issues • Review any needed follow-up • Review indications for return to treatment

From Group for the Advancement of Psychiatry (GAP) Committee on Child Psychiatry. *The Process of Child Therapy*. New York: Brunner, Mazel, 1982, with permission.

reenacts a past relationship and transfers it to the present relationship with you. Be aware that transference reactions will occur with the child as well as with his or her parents or guardians. Transference may be positive or negative (or, most commonly, a bit of both). Try to identify and work with transference early on. Retaining children and families in treatment is perhaps the biggest challenge—about 50% of children who begin treatment drop out before the therapy is successfully completed. This may be most common with the most severely ill youth and families, where the patient and his or her family (or both) may have a basic difficulty with engagement and trust. Maintaining a collaborative relationship with the guardians is integral to treatment integrity for the child.

 TIP

What kind of credentials do you have? When asked this at the first meeting, it may feel like a vote of "no confidence" from the parents and youth you are meeting—especially if you are still in training. Be aware that many parents (or sophisticated adolescents) are concerned about whether they can be understood and helped. Try a response to that basic issue. "I'm a _____ (e.g., resident, fellow, faculty, etc.) here at _____ (name of clinic or hospital). Are you concerned about my ability to help you?"

Other key issues to be aware of in the engagement period include empathic connection (recognizing and identifying with the patient's feelings), countertransference (the therapist's own feelings toward the patient and family), and appropriate therapeutic distance (how much or little to let a family know about you and how clear you are about the boundaries of the therapy). Working with children and youth can be quite complicated, as the therapist must be aware of and manage all of the issues of the child, as well as those of the parents.

Countertransference refers to the whole range of emotions that you may feel toward your patient (or his or her family), whether positive or negative. Novice interviewers have a tendency to try to suppress or ignore such feelings, especially when they are negative. Don't. These countertransference feelings represent some of the most clinically valuable material available to you. Whatever feelings your patient (or his or her family) elicits in you are feelings she probably elicits in most other people she encounters in her life. Knowing this can give you powerful insight into the nature of her problems.

Problem analysis is the stage in therapy where the issues to be addressed in therapy are identified. The parents and child will be helpful in identifying the problem list of issues they are motivated to change.

Developing an explanation of the problem is included in the "feedback session" to parents and youth. It outlines your understanding of the problem(s) and your recommendations for types of treatment. Ideally, an agreed upon treatment plan will result.

Establishing and implementing the formula for change is what is typically understood as the "therapy." It includes the sessions with the child, adolescent, family or group that are focused on working on the problems identified. Although there may be many theoretical bases and types of treatment, the *collaborative work for adaptive change*, with the ongoing assessment and readjustment of the therapy as needed, is key to all treatment modalities.

Termination is the portion of the therapy that prepares the child and family for ending the treatment. Sometimes, premature termination or "dropping out" will prohibit this. However, even in brief therapy (or unanticipated abbreviated therapy), a review of progress and any needed follow-up is essential.

TIP

The child or adolescent is typically brought by adults for treatment. Many times the identified child patient does not want to be there. He may feel that he is being punished or find it embarrassing to be brought for treatment with a "shrink." Address the resistance to treatment directly with the child and parent. For example, "You seem like you really don't want to be here. Is there something we can do together to make it more comfortable?" Children will often engage with the use of toys. Adolescents may wish to draw as they talk.

KEY POINT

Consent is a process by which a patient formally agrees to an evaluation or treatment. Informed consent for treatment with medication or psychotherapy can only be provided by adults that are legal guardians. However, assent (by minors) is also essential to the treatment process. In some states, minors can consent to psychotherapy without their parents' consent. Although this may occasionally be indicated, in general family or guardian involvement in the psychotherapeutic process is crucial. The consent process for psychotherapy, as with pharmacotherapy, includes providing the reasons that you consider the treatment medically indicated (benefits), as well as any potential risks (including the time and expense involved). Having both the minor patient and legal guardians maximally involved in understanding and consenting (as well as collaborating) is usually key to successful treatment.

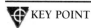 KEY POINT

Confidentiality is one of the primary tenets of psychotherapy. However, there are times when confidentiality must be broken. Inform children, youth, and parents/guardians of the confidentiality rules—that information discussed will be kept private unless there is risk to the youngster involved. The risks would include concern of abuse or neglect, issues of dangerousness (suicidality or homicidality), and serious risk-taking behaviors (drug use, running away, and potentially unsafe sexual practices). Inform the youth that you will help her talk to her parents about these issues if they come up. The fact that you inform the youth up front about the "rules," will help her maintain trust, even if you do need to help her tell her parents (or inform her that you are going to tell her parents) about these issues.

CLINICAL VIGNETTE

A 16-year-old girl has been discharged from her third psychiatric hospitalization for cutting and suicidality. She has left her prior therapist in favor of starting at a new clinic (for unclear reasons). A second-year child and adolescent psychiatry resident is meeting the patient for the intake interview.

> *Interviewer:*   *You have been in outpatient treatment before. Tell me, why did you decide to change clinics?*

Patient:	*My last therapist was such a jerk. I really don't think she knew what she was doing. How long have you been a psychiatrist?*
Interviewer:	*(Immediately feeling defensive.) Well, I am a second year child psychiatry resident.*
Patient:	*A resident! They had residents at the hospital and they never know what to do with me. Even the attendings are stumped. How many chronically suicidal adolescents have you treated . . . and did they live?*
Interviewer:	*(Increasingly uncomfortable and caught off guard). Well, I have treated a number of suicidal adolescents.*
Patient:	*How many?*
Interviewer:	*(Regaining composure and suddenly aware of how suspicious and frightened the patient is). Are you concerned that I won't understand or be able to help you?*

The patient then became tearful. Her feelings of being abandoned and not lovable, with her defensive antagonistic, angry, distrustful and somewhat grandiose behaviors became more obvious, and could gradually be discussed.

Evidence-Based Psychotherapies (EBPs)

EBPs refer to psychosocial treatments for which systematic controlled studies have established efficacy. The American Psychological Association has defined EBPs as treatments that have 1) randomized controlled research; 2) research designs with adequate sample size and defined study populations, 3) independent replication, and 4) taken into account feasibility, generalizability, cost and benefit. EBPs may be effective for depression, OCD, anxiety disorders, PTSD, and conduct problems. A summary of EBPs used in child and adolescent psychiatry is found in Table 25.3.

 TIP

If a child or adolescent presents with a specific fear or phobia and you do not have expertise in desensitization or exposure and response prevention techniques, you may need to refer the child to a colleague who has this expertise. Get to know the types of therapies indicated for presenting disorders and

TABLE 25.3. Examples of Evidence-based Psychotherapies

Psychiatric Problem	Evidence-based Psychotherapies	Developers
Anxiety	Coping cat Coping koala Family anxiety management	Kendall Barrett Dadds
OCD	CBT for OCD	March
Depression	CBT for depression IPT-A Primary and secondary control enhancement training Adolescent coping with depression	Asarnow, Stark Mufson et al. Weisz Clarke
ADHD	DCP STP	Barkley Pelham
Conduct disorder	PSST and PMT for conduct disorder MST Anger control training with stress inoculation Anger coping program Behavior parent training for youth with conduct problems Incredible years BASIC parent training program	Kazdin Henggeler Feindler Lochman Patterson Webster-Stratton
ODD	Parent—child interaction therapy for oppositional children DCP	Hood Barkley
Borderline personality disorder	DBT	Linehan (see Katz in bibliography)
SUD	MST	Henggeler

OCD, obsessive—compulsive disorder; CBT, cognitive-behavioral therapy; IPT-A, interpersonal psychotherapy for depressed adolescents; ADHD, attention deficit hyperactivity disorder; DCP, defiant children program; STP, summer treatment program; PSST, problem-solving skills training; PMT, parent management training; MST, multisystemic therapy; ODD, oppositional defiant disorder; DBT, dialectical behavior therapy; SUD, substance use disorders.

the individuals in your community to whom you may refer. Additionally, consider continued "tooling"—learning a variety of therapeutic techniques not only during your residency, but continuing to gain clinical skills through seminars and supervision to be proficient at a variety of therapeutic techniques.

WORKING WITH FAMILIES

Accurate psychiatric assessment and effective treatment of an individual child must involve an examination of family process. Family process refers to the repetitive patterns of interaction between members. Principles of family process are based on common patterns of family interactions. All families develop certain patterns of interaction—some may be adaptive and a source of family strength to be enhanced. Others may be maladaptive and the source of intervention.

Types of maladaptive or pathological family dynamics include:

- Powerful nonverbal communication that seeks to cut off real discussions of issues.
- Families that tend to maintain homeostasis, even when repetitive patterns are (or become as children develop) dysfunctional.
- Resistance of self-differentiation of family members.
- Enmeshment in which members are overconcerned or overinvolved in each other's lives. Boundaries in the family may be diffuse.
- Overly rigid boundaries that lead to disengagement of family members and little sense of family loyalty or unity.
- Triangulation of family dynamics, in which two family members unite against another family member.
- Family members may have an inability to manage stressful emotions and use the identified patient as the focus for all family angst or pathology.
- Families will try to include treating clinicians into their family "dance." At times, the clinician can contribute to maladaptive family dynamics by colluding with parents in a maladaptive manner of understanding and behaving toward their child.

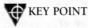 KEY POINT

The "identified patient" may be the individual that the family has identified as the "problem." However, often the family system itself may be dysfunctional, with the child's behavior a manifestation of that dysfunction. It is essential to have an assessment of family functioning (even if the child's family is a nontraditional family—grandparents, foster parents, or others). Be sure to have a family evaluation as part and parcel of all evaluations and family intervention included in the treatment process.

The Family Assessment

There are a number of theoretical approaches to assessing and treating families. The typical family assessment includes both a structured portion, as well as a more unstructured time. Construction of a family genogram is a common technique for assessing family function and understanding a family's history and patterns. The genogram maps out how family members are biologically and legally related one to another from one generation to the next. Typically, genograms start with the child's grandparents or great grandparents and add all subsequent family members. Any psychiatric, school, legal, substance use or other illnesses and suicides or other illnesses can be added next to each family member's circle (for females) or square (for males), so that it includes a family history of illness as well as a family history of interactions.

Another useful technique in assessing families is to get the entire family together to talk about a "typical day." You may ascertain when family members wake up, how they manage to get organized and out of the house in the morning, who is in charge of what, and when they are together (or not together). Ask about who sleeps where. Also ask about what each member likes about the family, and if they could change something about their family, what it would be. Including even little ones (the 4-year-old is often the one that "spills the beans" about dysfunctional family secrets) gives a good overall sense of the family's strengths, vulnerabilities, and areas of need.

Assessing parental skills is another valuable tool in the assessment of the family. Behavioral interventions (such as sticker charts and other rewards for positive behaviors) may be quite useful in treating behavior disorders in children. Utilizing a functional analysis of problem behaviors (triggers for when they occur, what makes them better, what makes them worse, how are they managed) may help generate a simple and easily implemented behavior plan. The hope is to decrease high emotion (yelling) and optimize positive reinforcement skills toward positive child behaviors. This decreases the conflict in the home and minimizes the negative attribution ("bad" boy) toward the child. I recommend to families that they focus on positive reinforcement (stickers, rewards, praise, privileges) of appropriate behaviors, using time-out from fun activities when the behavior is maladaptive or unsafe. Parent management training (PMT) is an evidence-based treatment for training parents to work with children with conduct issues in a consistent manner utilizing proven behavioral techniques. This may be the most effective single treatment for the child or adolescent with conduct disorder in the absence of more complex psychiatric pathology.

Family Therapy

Although families should be involved in almost all therapies for children and youth in some manner, at times treatment intervention is most effectively centered on the family dynamics. There are a number of family therapy perspectives that inform the type of family intervention utilized.

Common indications for family evaluation and intervention are the presence of serious medical conditions or psychiatric disorders, the passing of important life-cycle transitions and events, and failure of nonfamily therapy–oriented psychological or medical treatments. At times, the assessment will identify serious substance abuse or mental health issues in a parent which require referral and treatment. Family therapy may be useful in helping the family cope with the parent's illness. However, it is essential to avoid inadvertently allowing the child to be in a caretaker role for a parent. If parental psychopathology endangers the child, protective services may need to be involved.

Although child and adolescent psychiatrists often do a great deal of psychoeducation with parents, family therapy may not be an area of expertise. Every clinician should develop techniques for family assessment, engaging the family in the understanding and treatment of the child, and an awareness of when family therapy needs to be a primary focus of the treatment of an individual child or adolescent. Children or adolescents with serious medical or psychiatric disorders will require a thorough family evaluation and intervention. If you do not have expertise in family therapy, identify resources that can provide this. I recommend having several clinicians with whom you gain a good working relationship for cross-referral within a clinic or in the community.

Splitting treatment can be quite effective if there is good communication among clinicians regarding the focus of the treatment. Poor communication among several providers invites splitting or fragmentation of treatment.

SUMMARY

Psychosocial treatments are indicated for almost all psychiatric disorders affecting children and adolescents. First, provide a thorough assessment of child and family functioning. Identify both strengths and weaknesses of the child and family. Use this information to formulate an individualized treatment program that takes into account the level of intensity of intervention required, the type(s) of therapies indicated, and the involvement of the family in the therapeutic process. Systems of care, wrap-around services, and in-home interventions are supports that may be helpful for families and children with functionally disabling symptoms. The child and adolescent psychiatrist formulates an individual case, develops skills at identifying the appropriate interventions for an individual child and family, and works collaboratively within a broader system of care to ensure that the child or adolescent receives the most integrated and effective treatment possible.

Psychoeducational Interventions

Essential Concepts
- The Individuals with Disabilities Act (IDEA) mandates that all children who need special services receive them in the least restrictive appropriate environment.
- Children who receive special education services have an Individualized Educational Plan (IEP) which specifies the type of special services required and to be provided to the child.
- There is a full range of modifications within the educational system for children with special needs, depending on the severity, chronicity, and ability of the child to learn in each setting.
- In working within the school setting, the child and adolescent psychiatrist must understand the school culture and work collaboratively with multidisciplinary school personnel, the student, parents, primary care physician, and any outpatient treaters to help the school set up an appropriate educational plan for the student.

Education is not the filling of a pail but the lighting of a fire.

—W. B. Yeats

GENERAL PRINCIPLES AND CLINICAL CONSIDERATIONS

An estimated 3 to 10% of children in public school demonstrate significant and impairing psychopathology. Additionally, between 70 and 80% of children who receive mental health services receive them in schools. For many of these children, school is their only mental health resource. Schools are required by law to educate children and youth. Emotional, behavioral, and learning disorders that interfere with that education become the purview of schools via special education or Section 504 services.

For most children, school is a stabilizing part of their lives. They gain self-esteem and a feeling of self-efficacy through learning, socializing, sports and games, and a positive relationship with their teachers, the significant adults outside of the home. For children and adolescents with psychiatric and learning disorders, however, school may be a very negative place, where they feel at a loss as to how to make and keep friends, pay attention, control their behavior, or keep up with their work. Understanding how children function at home, as well as how they function at school, is important in understanding the nature of the emotional problems and the environmental triggers that exacerbate or ameliorate them.

Children spend a great deal of time in schools. Although all schools have similar mandates and requirements, each school has its own unique character and culture. Children who may thrive in one school environment may struggle in another. It is extremely gratifying to work in the school setting as part of a team that helps a youngster who is troubled or troubling to be more successful. To do so, you must understand some of the basic laws and requirements, as well as types of services that may be provided in the school. Additionally, going into the school culture, you must always be ready to learn—about the unique aspects of the school, the strengths and areas of weakness, resource availability, and how to negotiate successfully within the educational system.

⊕ KEY POINT

A child and adolescent psychiatrist may provide support to a school in a myriad of ways:

- Direct treatment within the school (school-based clinic model)
- School-based evaluations and recommendations for individual students who have been identified as having difficulties
- Consultation—providing expert opinion to the school with regard to programming, curriculum, or services
- Collaboration—ongoing contact with school, student, etc. in the joint process of improving outcome

---

Practical Aspects of Working in Schools: IDEA vs. Section 504 (Table 26.1)

The Individuals with Disabilities Education Act (IDEA) and Section 504 of the Rehabilitation Act of 1973 allow for special services for children with special needs. IDEA is a

TABLE 26.1. Comparison of IDEA vs. Section 504 Services and Regulations

IDEA	Section 504
All school-aged children who have a disabling qualifying condition (autism, learning disability, speech or language impairment, emotional disturbance, traumatic brain injury, visual impairment, hearing impairment, deafness, mental retardation, deaf-blindness, multiple disabilities, orthopedic impairment, and other health impairments)	Individuals who meet the definition of qualified "handicapped" person—having a physical or mental impairment that substantially limits a major life activity (walking, seeing, hearing, speaking, breathing, learning, working, caring for oneself, performing manual tasks)
Disability must adversely affect educational performance	Does not require special education eligibility
Evaluation—full, comprehensive evaluation by multidisciplinary team	Evaluation draws on information from a variety of sources
Requires informed and written consent	Does not require consent of parents, only notice
Requires reevaluation at least once every 3 years	"Periodic" reevaluation required
Provides for independent evaluation at district expense if parents disagree with first evaluation	No provision for independent evaluation at school's expense
Reevaluation not required before a significant change in placement	Reevaluation required before a significant change in placement
Requires an individualized educational program (IEP) with at least annual review	Does not require an IEP, but does require a plan

218

Participants required at IEP meeting include parents, general education teacher, special education teacher, school administrator, psychologist/person to interpret evaluation results, the child (if appropriate)	Participants not mandated
Appropriate education is program designed to provide "educational benefit"	Appropriate education means education "comparable" to that of nondisabled peers
Placement may be in any combination of special education and general education classrooms	Placement usually in general education classroom
Related services, if required	Related services, if needed
Impartial hearings for parents who disagree with identification, evaluation, or placement of student	Impartial hearings for parents who disagree with identification, evaluation, or placement of student
Requires written consent	No consent requirement
Delineates specific procedures	Parent has opportunity to participate and be represented by counsel
Hearing Officer appointed by impartial appointee	Hearing Officer usually appointed by school
Provides "stay-put" provision until all proceedings are resolved	No "stay-put" provisions
Parents must receive 10-day notice prior to any change in placement	No requirement of days notice prior to change of placement
Enforced by U.S. Department of Education, Office of Special Education	Enforced by U.S. Department of Education, Office of Civil Rights

federal law that guarantees special education and related services for those students who meet the criteria for eligibility. Every child with a disability is entitled to a free appropriate education (FAPE) designed to meet his or her individual needs.

Some children with special needs are not served under IDEA but are served under Section 504. This is a civil rights law that prohibits discrimination on the basis of disabling conditions. If a child is deemed to have a mental or physical impairment that affects a major life function (but the impairment does not have a significant adverse effect on educational performance), he or she is eligible for Section 504 services. Some families prefer to have their children receive services under Section 504, because they are not then "labeled" as special education students.

Special Education Services

Children are assessed to have a disability via individualized evaluation examining all aspects of a potential disability. To qualify for special educational services, a child must have a handicapping condition that interferes with educational performance. At-risk infants and toddlers with developmental delays are eligible for services. School services for children with special needs begin at the age of 3.

There are 13 categories of disability specified under IDEA (as noted in Table 26.1). The ones typically relevant to mental health professionals include autism (any autism-spectrum disorder), emotional disturbance (ED), and other health impairment (often used for attention deficit hyperactivity disorder, ADHD). There are approximately 5.5 million children with disabilities who receive special education services in the United States.

ED is defined as a condition that exhibits one or more of the following characteristics over a long period of time and to a marked degree and that adversely affect a child's educational performance:

- An inability to learn that cannot be explained by intellectual, sensory, or health factors
- An inability to build or maintain satisfactory interpersonal relationships with peers and teachers
- Inappropriate types of behaviors or feelings under normal circumstances

- A general pervasive mood of unhappiness or depression
- A tendency to develop physical symptoms or fears associated with personal or school problems

Psychiatric Evaluations Within the School Setting

Child and adolescent psychiatrists may be requested to provide a psychiatric evaluation for a school system. This is often to assess a child or adolescent who is demonstrating significant emotional and/or behavioral difficulties that are disruptive to the other children and for whom the school personnel feel at a loss as to how to be helpful. Often, there have been a number of interventions already tried.

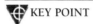 KEY POINT

There is a new vocabulary to learn when you work with schools. You have already learned IDEA, Section 504, and FAPE. Although states vary in some of the acronyms, these are the basics that are fairly widely used:

PPT (Planning and Placement Team) or IEP Meeting—PPT meetings (also called IEP meetings) are those meetings that are held with appropriate membership (regular education teacher, special education teacher, school administrator, and parent, at minimum) to make any legally binding decisions and plans about a child's school curriculum that varies from the standard curriculum.

IEP—Individualized Educational Plan. This is the plan that includes goals and objectives, and specifies the hours of service provided and by whom they will be provided for any child who receives special education services.

IEP Meeting—(also called a Planning and Placement Team or PPT meeting). Makes any legally binding decisions and plans about a child's school curriculum that varies from the standard curriculum.

LEA—Local Educational Agency. This is typically the town or district that funds the educational services for the child.

Procedural Safeguards—must be given to the legal guardians at key points in the educational process. The Safeguards outline the legal rights of the family/legal guardians regarding the educational process and include specifications about evaluations, prior written notice of meetings and changes in an educational plan, parental consent, child's school placement, mediation, due process, and appeals process.

 KEY POINT

Legal and Ethical Aspects of the Consultation

1. Parents may refuse direct interaction between the psychiatrist and their child. Parents must consent to direct assessment (although not indirect consultation to school personnel).
2. Risk assessment—in situations of acute suicidality or homicidality, the consultant may facilitate appropriate emergency treatment.
3. Suspected abuse—school personnel and medical personnel both have the obligation to report.

 TIP

I recommend setting aside at least 2½ to 3 hours for a school-related evaluation. I use the following format to most efficiently gain the information required for a thorough psychiatric evaluation in the school setting. For practicalities and convenience, the schedule may change to suit the situation.

1. Clarify guardian consent, understanding of the nature of the consult, and consultation question.
2. Request to have school records sent to you ahead of time, so that you can review—prior testing, behavior plans, PPT minutes, and the IEP (if the child has already been designated eligible for special education services) are all documents that you will find helpful.
3. 30 minutes: Meet with school personnel who know the child. Get details about the major difficulties observed, what interventions have been tried and how they worked, and strengths of the child.
4. 60 minutes: Parent interview—I encourage both parents to come (even if they are divorced). Review the history: developmental, family, medical, psychiatric and diagnostic symptom review. What is the parental view of their child's difficulties and strengths—at home and at school? What do the parents feel would be helpful? Get Release of Information forms signed for primary care physician and any mental health treaters.
5. 60+ minutes: The student interview—if the child is young, a classroom observation may be indicated (about 30 minutes). Observe adaptive and maladaptive behavior. Meet individually with the child for a fairly standard mental status examination, which usually includes drawing, talking, and/or playing, depending on the age and interests of the

child. Include diagnostic and risk assessment questions (abuse, neglect, substance use, homicidality, suicidality) as for all psychiatric assessments. What does the child like to do, how does she feel about school, what problems does she feel interfere with school behavior?

6. Wrap-up—if time and schedules permit, I typically meet with school personnel to review the day and preliminary thoughts. Any further information or clarification about the child is gathered. Schedule the PPT meeting (usually about 2 weeks later).

7. After leaving—call other sources of information (primary care physician, mental health treaters, or others) and write up the report. Fax the report to the school (if they requested the evaluation) first. Then review the findings with the parents (ideally in person, but sometimes over the phone) prior to the PPT. Go to the PPT meeting to verbally detail findings and recommendations, and work with the Team in formulating a plan.

The School Evaluation Report:

- Identifying information (name of student, date of birth, date of assessment, sources of information
- Reason for evaluation and referral questions
- History of present difficulties
- Pertinent history: developmental, medical, psychiatric, school
- Interview of the child: mental status examination (and observation, if applicable)
- Diagnosis
- Formulation
- Educational recommendations (as specific as possible about the components of an educational plan that would be expected to improve functioning)
  - Special education eligibility discussion (e.g., emotional disturbance, other health impaired, etc.)
  - Need for further assessment—cognitive and academic testing, speech and language, OT, etc.
  - Type of classroom setting—number, student-teacher ratios, special tutoring or resource room support, paraprofessional assistance, etc.
  - Behavioral plans (from functional assessment of behaviors)
  - Other services—social work or other in-school mental health support, social skills groups, modified PE, etc.
  - Other recommendations—school–parent interface, how the outpatient team may be involved, special school activities for self-esteem or relationship building

- Noneducational recommendations about treatment or other services the family may implement that are not directly related to the school responsibility to educate the student

---

CLINICAL VIGNETTE

The following is the diagnosis, formulation, and educational recommendations sections of a psychiatric school evaluation.

Diagnosis:

Axis I:	Bipolar disorder
	Attention deficit hyperactivity disorder, combined type
	Oppositional-defiant disorder
Axis II:	Deferred
Axis III:	No active medical conditions
Axis IV:	Educational and social supports
Axis V:	Global assessment of functioning = 50

Formulation

John Smith is a 12-year-old regular education student with a history of difficulties with distractibility and inattention, intermittent temper outbursts, and periods of mood instability which have interfered with social relationships and his ability to make expected gains academically. John's present and prior psychological testing suggests that he is a bright boy with many cognitive skills and assets. "Cognitive strengths include a well-developed fund of knowledge, excellent mental computational skills and exceptional visual-motor construction ability. Cognitive challenges include inconsistent performance on grapho-motor tasks, a relative weakness in auditory attention and working memory, challenges with executive functioning and inconsistent access to memory skills."

Despite his considerable talents in many areas, John is not doing well academically and socially. John has biological vulnerabilities in the areas of attentional issues, a biologically based mood disorder, and difficulties with executive functioning that impair his judgment and ability to control his impulses. At a developmental time when he should be increasingly motivated by skill acquisition and increasingly interested in peer relationships, group affiliations, and out-of-family adult role models, John is shutting himself off from many of these opportunities. John presents with very fragile self-esteem and exquisite sensitivity to perceived rejection or embarrassment. John seems to perceive the world as a menacing, unfair, and rejecting place, where he is constantly in jeopardy of humiliation. This world view leaves him hypersensitive to any perceived criticism, often misperceiving neutral or mildly negative interactions as true affronts to his self-esteem. His fear of feeling inadequate is so great at present that he often cannot tolerate a paper being examined and corrected.

John has symptoms that meet diagnostic criteria for ADHD (difficulties with sustained attention, distractibility) and oppositional-defiant disorder (constant rejection of limits and refusal to cooperate). However, the more concerning issue at this point for John is his high level of emotional distress. His mood swings, high levels of anger, grandiosity, misperceptions and suspiciousness, extreme reactivity, and very poor self-concept indicate a mood disorder (bipolar disorder). Despite his desperate efforts to hide his unhappiness, it pervades his behavior, frequently presenting as oppositionality, frustration, or anger.

A key issue in programming academically for John is engagement. At the present time, he is quite defensive and mistrustful, and his work productivity is minimal. An academic environment with minimal stimulation and a high degree of structure, which works well for simple ADHD with oppositionality, has not been particularly successful for John. For him, refusal to do work is frequently an interpersonal issue (fear of not doing it perfectly, fear of embarrassment). Helping John feel in control, such that he does not feel excessively vulnerable, while helping him contain his acting out (disruptive, uncooperative) behaviors and gaining self-esteem through genuine effort, rather than product only, will likely be key.

John has many strengths. He can be engagable and engaging. He has a number of interests. He is athletic and bright. He is creative, interesting, and fun. He wants to be successful. He desperately craves acceptance and relationships with his peers and adults. He has responded very positively to a home tutor who works closely with John in a nonconfrontive manner and has been able to help John engage and learn the material.

Recommendations

Educational Recommendations

1. It is recommended that the Planning and Placement Team review the criteria for eligibility for special education services, under the exceptionality of Emotional Disturbance.

John has demonstrated an inability to build and maintain satisfactory interpersonal relationships with peers and teachers, inappropriate behaviors and feelings under normal circumstances, and a general pervasive mood of unhappiness for the academic year, or longer.

2. The initial task is to help John improve his productivity (allow himself to engage in the academic work). Thus, a focus on effort, rather than product, will be essential. The following interventions are recommended:

   - A consistent behavior management plan between home and school, which provides for consistency of expectations and continuity of rewards and consequences. John should be optimally engaged to ensure "buy-in" on his part; additionally, parents, outpatient treater, and school personnel should be involved.

   - Goal of appropriate academic behavior (doing work)— It is recommended that John receive a reward (computer time or other activity) after a brief time of genuine academic effort, with the effort time expected to gradually increase as John is able to do his work.

   - Goal of appropriate social behavior (not being disruptive or disrespectful)—A separate reward (positive time with teacher, counselor, mentor, etc.) for appropriate classroom behavior, to begin with brief times and increased as he masters this, is recommended.

   - Goal of engagement—John may respond positively to extra "special" responsibilities that highlight his strengths (messages to the office, computer assistance, public presentations, or "managing" something), helping him to feel special, valued, and needed, and allowing him to form meaningful relationships with school personnel.

   - The present pattern of severe work refusal and disruptive behaviors in the classroom suggests that this is a maladaptive pattern that will require a very different educational approach. John has done well at home with a tutor in a quiet setting. Having a one-to-one tutor out of the classroom for academic subjects to break the maladaptive pattern, help John engage, catch up in his learning, and experience success academically and interpersonally is recommended. The tutor will need to be an individual who understands and is able to work empathically with John's confrontive style. This plan should be tried, with John involved in working out the details. If it is successful, the plan should continue uninterrupted with a "re-integration" plan (slowly starting to get back into resource room and other classes as he is ready).

- Special educational support (direct and indirect) to help with curriculum development, provide oversight to the academic work, help with organizational skills, and ensure consistent implementation of the behavior plan is recommended.
- Modifications for ADHD—preferential seating, cuing, monitoring, and teaching organizational skills are recommended for John.
- Work volume should be minimized, when possible, to decrease the frustration and overwhelming aspects of the tasks for John. Concept acquisition and effort should be rewarded.
- Modifications for learning issues—A specific organizational skill development plan (organizational checklists, homework notebook, etc.) is recommended. Developing computer and word processing skills may be particularly helpful to John in getting his thoughts onto paper effectively.
- Social skills development—It is recommended that John receive in-school counseling at least 30 minutes weekly for support, and problem-solving and coping skills work. A small social skills group (lunch group or other) to help John gain the skills he needs socially for acceptance and friendships is recommended.
- Lunch in a quiet place with a few other students or teachers, as appropriate.
- Regular communication and consensus among the school personnel, John's parents, and outpatient mental health treater (Dr. Jones) will be essential to his comfort level in school, to consistent and unified behavioral management planning and implementation, and to ensure that any difficulties are promptly and effectively addressed. It is recommended that a meeting to review John's progress and the success of a new program occur within 1 to 2 months after it is implemented, for early evaluation and modification of the plan, as appropriate.

3. If John is unable to make academic and social progress within the public school setting, he will require a special educational placement in a day school with expertise and a full therapeutic curriculum for working with students with emotional, attentional, and behavioral difficulties.

TIP

Students are invited to the IEP meetings, and may be in attendance. Word your findings in lay language that is nonjudgmental and matter of fact. If the student is there, be sure to talk to him directly about findings and engage him in the solution. Although initially uncomfortable, having the student in the meeting frequently helps him feel more engaged in the plan and less as though a plan is being "done to him" if the discussion is sensitive, respectful, and highlights strengths as well as difficulties.

Consultations to Systems of Care

> **Essential Concepts**
> - Clarification of the role of the consultant is essential to successful consultation to any system.
> - As a consultant, address each of the "Who, What, Where, When, Why, How?" questions.
> - Consultations occur to many systems and in many venues. Consultations to systems require a broad perspective and expertise about how the system works and how to negotiate within each system.
> - Intervening in disasters is a systems-based consultation that provides services to optimize outcomes for a large number of traumatized children and families.

GENERAL PRINCIPLES AND CLINICAL CONSIDERATIONS

The consultation role is very different from a treatment role. Child and adolescent psychiatrists may consult to many different systems: pediatric inpatient, outpatient, and specialty services, courts, schools, mental health service agencies, disaster victims and service providers, policy-makers, the media, and many others. Although there are many unique aspects of consultation to a specific system, there are also many similarities. The present chapter will set a framework for systems-based consultations, with special attention to consultation-liaison to pediatrics, court-ordered consultations, systems consultations to schools and service agencies, and crisis consultation after a disaster.

Framework for Consultations

The clearer roles, responsibilities, and expectations are prior to a consultation, the more satisfied all will be with the consultant's involvement and the more helpful the recommendations will be.

1. **WHO? The Consultee and Confidentiality Parameters**
   a. *Who* is requesting the consultation? What is the system involved?
   b. Clarify the multidisciplinary staff that may be affected by the consultation—clarify their goals and ensure their input and involvement.
   c. Clarify confidentiality, with whom the consultant will interact, informed consent around consultant interactions (if relevant), and nature of the recommendations (written report, verbal, case conference, etc.) and with whom it will be shared.

2. **WHAT? Clarification of the Consultation Question and Wishes/Needs of the Consultee**
   a. What are the consultation questions? Seek to understand the consultee's concerns and help focus the consultation question.
   b. Are the goals for the consultation realistic? Success depends on realistic expectations and a shared consensus about the nature of the problem.
   c. Clarify the role of the consultant—whether the consultation is direct (direct observation/assessment of an individual child with recommendations) or indirect (consultation to treaters or personnel only).
   d. Clarify (if possible) if the request is for a "hired gun" vs. an impartial consultant.

3. **WHERE? Where will the consultation take place?**
   a. Choose the location that is most convenient
   b. Be sure that you are "in the mix" with the personnel, students, patients, etc. to whom you are providing the consultation.

4. **WHEN? What is the time frame to complete the consultation?**
   a. Is there time to complete the consultation requested?

5. **WHY? Why is the request for consultation being made at this time?**
   a. Sometimes the ostensible reason for the request covers a "hidden agenda," such as staffing issues, conflict among staff, difficult parents, or others.

6. **HOW? How will the consultation proceed?**
   a. How much of the workup has been done before proceeding with the consultation?
   b. How will the consultant get the information needed to proceed with the consultation?
   c. How will the results of the consultation be communicated?

Models of Consultation-Liaison to Pediatricians

Several models of consultation-liaison have been developed in response to the kinds of consultations requested by pediatricians and to the kinds of psychological reactions prominent in hospitalized pediatric patients and their families.

1. Anticipatory Model—this is a consultation to a child and family in anticipation of a difficult procedure. Pretreatment psychiatric consultation to assess the strengths and vulnerabilities of the family and to prepare the child and family accordingly may be very helpful. This process may help avert serious psychological reactions or ensure that psychiatric support is in place if or when they occur.
2. Case Finding Model—this includes liaison work—regular ward meetings with pediatric and nursing staff that enhance the functioning of the unit and help with early identification of patients at risk. This model may encompass the (often not specifically requested) identification of staff communication or systems and relational issues to be addressed.
3. Education and Training Model—training for pediatricians, pediatric house-staff, nurses, and collaborative case conferences and didactics enhance the effectiveness of all the treaters of the children and families.
4. Emergency Response Model—this model ensures consultation coverage for children and adolescents in acute crisis. The consultation request is typically urgent, such as how to manage an acutely upset, aggressive, or suicidal patient on the wards.
5. Continuing and Collaborative Care Model—this is best suited for children with recurring or chronic medical illnesses and may occur in inpatient or outpatient settings, or both.

Consultation to the Courts

Court-ordered consultations may include psychiatric assessments of children and youth who have committed crimes (such as competency to stand trial and "amenability to treatment" evaluations), custody evaluations, or expert witness testimony.

Juvenile Court. Mental health professionals are called on by the juvenile court to perform evaluations, make treatment and program recommendations, and provide consultation and expert testimony. Youth who have been accused of committing a crime are often released to the custody of a parent or guardian unless a judge deems detention necessary for the protection of the community or is otherwise in the child's best interest. The juvenile delinquency proceeding includes the "adjudication hearing" (trial). If the youth is found guilty, he is "adjudicated" (convicted). If there has been adjudication, the case proceeds to the "dispositional" (sentencing) phase. At the preadjudicatory and postadjudicatory stages of a juvenile delinquency proceeding, the need for treatment, appropriate type of treatment, and likelihood of benefit from treatment are questions posed to mental health treaters. Issues of competency to stand trial are usually more relevant for older youth who have been referred to the adult criminal court due to the youth's age, seriousness, or chronicity of offenses.

 TIP

For consultations to the juvenile justice system, review the who, what, where, when, why, and how questions. Clarify for yourself, the youth and family, and the court what the nature of confidentiality is. In general, court-ordered evaluations have *no* confidentiality, and the youth needs to be informed of that (what he or she says may end up in your report to the court).

Custody Consultations.

Most divorcing parents make their own custody arrangements. About 25% of divorces experience substantial or intense conflict over custody. Contested custody occurs in about 5 to 8% of parental divorces. Most of these cases settle during the trial, but for 1.5% of families, the judge determines the custody or visitation issue.

Mental health professionals who have a confidential individual therapeutic relationship with a child typically do not participate in the custody evaluations (as this jeopardizes the confidential and neutral relationship). Although a parent can subpoena a therapist, usually the therapeutic confidentiality will be honored.

Consultation to the court in the matter of child custody may be a prolonged and bitter dispute. Consultants again need to review the "who, what, where, when, why, and how" questions of the consultation. In particular, is the child and adolescent psychiatrist impartial (hired by the court for the purpose of the evaluation) or hired by one of the parents as an expert witness for his or her case. The typical questions posed by the court for the child and adolescent psychiatrist expert witness include:

- With whom should the child live?
- Which parent should have legal decision-making authority regarding education, medical decisions, religion, financial support, vacations, and so forth?
- How can the opportunities for the child to maintain a useful and sound relationship with both parents be optimized?

Court-ordered evaluations are not confidential. Ensure knowledge of this, and get signed consent forms to talk to any outside treaters or agencies.

 TIP

Testifying in court may seem particularly daunting to the novice. The primary issues to consider are as follows: 1) The reason you are testifying in court (are you the expert witness who has reviewed evidence or done an evaluation on which you are reporting, are you subpoenaed for a child abuse or state custody issue, etc.?; 2) What your opinion actually is (and why) distilled down to a conclusion that is understandable and in lay terms; 3) *You are not the one on trial.* Resist acting in a defensive, adversarial, or know-it-all manner. Be truthful, answer questions simply, and don't let yourself be flustered by an aggressive attorney. Your opinion is being requested because you have valuable information or expertise to offer the court that will help inform the judge or jury's decision. I recommend reviewing your findings and conclusions carefully with an attorney before you testify. Anticipate the issues beforehand so that you may address them appropriately when you are on the stand.

Systems-Based Consultation to Schools

Some school-based consultations are not focused on an individual child, but on the system. In particular, a variety of schools may find the expertise of a child and adolescent psychiatrist or other mental health professionals useful. This allows a venue in which to problem-solve a host of issues—overall behavioral management in the classroom, substance and mental health issues in the school, or "staffings" about specific children, with problem solving about recommended techniques for addressing emotional and behavioral issues of that child prior to requiring a formal assessment or plan. Table 27.1 outlines the components of a systems-based consultation.

◆ KEY POINT

Schools do not often request a systems consultation. However, if you consult to a school system, you may note recurrent issues and themes. For example, in one school to which
I consulted, there were a number of questions by teachers
and guidance staff about the marked increase in children
diagnosed with bipolar disorder, and how to deal with
them (and their families, who came to the school after visiting a website and demanded a number of services). Training in-services, "case conference" discussions, and reviewing some literature, as well as devising an overall strategy of
understanding (similarities and differences) and programming for children and youth with mood instability were very
helpful to the school staff.

TABLE 27.1. Components of a Systems-based Assessment

1. Assess the power structure, administration–teacher working
   relationship, school–central administration relationship, parental
   involvement, and strengths and weaknesses of communication
   channels, coping mechanisms (maladaptive such as scapegoating
   or more productive problem solving), resources, and morale.
2. Consultation questions often do not involve an interest in systems
   assessment—it is frequently threatening and requires a great
   deal of trust-building and empathy.
3. Ally with consultee
   a. Validate consultee perceptions
   b. Share anxiety
   c. Cultivate respect for everyone
4. Diminishing resistances
   a. Find each person's contribution
   b. Ask additional questions before posing a solution
   c. Status-equilibrating statements
5. Align consultee objectives
   a. Use consultee's own words
   b. Find where good intent went awry
   c. Help others see the child(ren) differently
   d. Appeal to shared values in posing solutions
   e. Build bridges between and beyond members of the existing
      system
   f. Reconsider underlying fears if consultees cannot work toward
      a solution

(Continued)

TABLE 27.1. **Components of a Systems-based Assessment**
(*continued*)

6. Act
   a. Expand the consultee's skills
   b. Identify one step up from the current situation and start solution plans there
   c. Identify individual timetables
   d. Move the system from reactive to proactive

Consultation to Systems of Care

Child and adolescent psychiatrists are called on to consult to a variety of systems that care for children and adolescents. Child welfare services in which children and adolescents may be cared for include foster care homes, group homes, youth shelters, domestic violence shelters, mentorship programs, or other systems of care.

When child service agencies are overwhelmed or faced with situations of crisis, they may call on mental health professionals for help. Quite often, these agencies have difficulty in articulating the type or degree of problem that they are having. First, the mental health consultant must help the requesting person or agency define the problem and refine the questions that they wish to have addressed. Second, the consultant must be clear about his or her role as a helper in the problem-solving process. The consultant must recognize the limits of his or her knowledge and power. Consultants should recognize that issues related to insight, unconscious motivation, and acting out may be encountered and dealt with in the consultation process. It is important not to become the individual therapist for those to whom you consult, but to identify and work with the issues that arise in a manner that may promote growth of the team. Finally, by taking the time to understand the culture of the consultation site through a naturalistic or ethnographic intervention, the consultant is better able to understand the point of view of the client. This allows the mental health consultant's knowledge of child psychiatry to be most useful to agency personnel, volunteers, and the children who are served by these programs. The typical consultation includes staff that have attempted to work out a difficulty and have not been successful. The first task of the consultant is to ascertain the type of help that is needed; it can be categorized into one of two types: (1) *clinical* consultation and (2) *programmatic* consultation.

Clinical consultation is usually related to an individual person, family, or group. Usually the consultant is asked to "reveal" information about the individual that will improve the agency's ability to serve the client. Most commonly, this is the "acting out" or rageful child or adolescent.

Programmatic consultation usually relates to the staff and programmatic curriculum of an agency. Programmatic consultation is directed toward broader organizational change with the goal of improving the care provided or services rendered. Identification of training needs, or providing useful training, education, and supervision may be a key aspect to programmatic consultation.

Crisis Consultations

After the terrorist attacks of 9/11 "disaster psychiatry" has become a more essential skill. Bombings, shootings, and violent crimes personally affect an increasing number of children and youth in the United States. It is estimated that 10% of all public schools experience one or more serious violent crimes (i.e., murder, rape or sexual battery, suicide, physical attack or fight with a weapon, or robbery) that were reported to local law enforcement officials during any school year (4% elementary, 19% middle school, 21% high school).

These startling statistics make it more essential that child and adolescent psychiatrists are able to intervene effectively in a crisis situation. I will focus on schools here, as that is the most common consultation venue for crisis-based intervention to a group.

Table 27.2 outlines the issues and elements of consultation to schools to prepare for and to intervene effectively in a crisis.

TABLE 27.2. Systems Consultation for Disaster Prevention and Intervention

1. School's Preparedness for a Disaster
   a. Safe School plans
   b. Schools vary widely in their preparedness to respond to a crisis
   c. Collaboration with law enforcement, community agencies, other mental health workers, school personnel, parents, students, etc. is essential for an effective crisis response plan that is flexible enough to be adapted to a variety of situations and uses as its foundation principles of developmental psychology, stress management, and crisis intervention

(Continued)

TABLE 27.2. Systems Consultation for Disaster Prevention and Intervention (*continued*)

2. Elements of Consultation
   a. Effective coordination of the elements of crisis response is fundamental—usually by administrative office of school
   b. Needs assessment—key school personnel, students, and parents
   c. Data gathering about nature and effect of crisis
   d. Support for crisis intervention workers is key
3. Direct Services
   a. Debriefing—individuals with shared experiences are brought together to discuss their personal reactions, through which mutual support may be derived.
   b. Critical Incident Stress Debriefing (CISD) by Mitchell is one model.
      i. Ventilation of intense emotions
      ii. Exploration of intense emotions
      iii. Group support
      iv. Initiation of the grief process within a supportive environment
      v. Reduction of the "fallacy of uniqueness"
      vi. Reassurance that intense emotions under such conditions are normal
      vii. Preparation for the continuation of the grief/stress process in the near future
      viii. Warning of possible emotional, cognitive, and physical symptoms
      ix. Education regarding normal and abnormal stress response syndromes
      x. Encouragement for continued group support or other professional assistance
      xi. Classroom meetings to help children talk on their own level about their experience, fears, perceptions, and reassurance of adults to care for them
      xii. Drawing, story telling, or story writing may be useful
      xiii. Early identification of PTSD symptoms
      xiv. A discussion of hope and reparations at age-appropriate level
      xv. Ensuring that children experience a unified adult concern and attendance to their safety which will help them with their fears, and letting parents know the usual manifestations in a child of that age and warning signs of need for further intervention.

(Continued)

TABLE 27.2. Systems Consultation for Disaster Prevention and Intervention (*continued*)

---

    xvi. Parent support, school personnel support, direct services, screening, and providing an atmosphere of understanding and support may also be needed

  c. School Personnel

    i. Teachers and school personnel will need to meet separately for support, debriefing, and education about dealing with the crisis with the children

    ii. Education about PTSD symptoms in children and adults and when professional help is needed, and stress relief

    iii. Education about maintaining an atmosphere of familiarity and routine for students

  d. Parents

    i. Group meetings with parents may be indicated

    ii. Review of event, support, brief didactics, question-and-answer, and advice on how to help themselves and child cope with disaster—when to seek professional help

  e. Media

    i. May be key to effective crisis response

    ii. May add to disruption by secondary trauma of graphic coverage, etc.

    iii. Interface with media and parents about how to monitor, limit, or support exposure to media coverage

    iv. Positive use of media for education about potential psychological response and community resources and assistance

  f. Recovery Environment

    i. The reaction of the greater community may enhance or disrupt recovery (secondary or "process trauma")

SUMMARY

The child and adolescent psychiatrist may serve a number of roles within the overall health and mental health service delivery system. Consultation to systems in which children and youth receive services is one of the ways to make a significant and positive impact. Seminars, readings, and active learning with a more experienced child and adolescent psychiatrist are all ways to gain and improve consultation skills.

APPENDICES

Essentials of the Child and Adolescent Psychiatric Evaluation/Report

1. Identifying information
   a. Age, sex, grade in school, with whom the child lives
   b. Referral source
   c. Sources of information (parents, teachers, pediatrician, child, etc.)
   d. Chief complaint or reason for referral (the chief complaint may differ between parent and child)
2. History of present illness
   a. Difficulties that prompted the evaluation
   b. Context in which problems occur
   c. Review of psychiatric symptoms
3. Past psychiatric history (THOMAS)
   a. **T**reatment (**H**ospitalizations, residential or day treatments, **O**utpatient)
   b. **M**edications—History and present psychotropic medication use
   c. **A**ttempts at **S**uicide or self-injurious behaviors
4. Medical history (MIDAS)
   a. Current **M**edications
   b. Medical **I**llnesses
   c. Primary care **D**octor
   d. **A**llergies
   e. **S**urgeries
5. Developmental and social history
   a. Pregnancy (including any medications, substances, major illness, or complications), delivery, and early infancy including temperament
   b. Developmental milestones and toilet training
   c. Educational history from preschool on (including any special services or special education)
   d. Social history (peer relationships, activities, sexual behavior, etc.)
   e. Electronics (use of Internet, video games, TV, movies—how much, what type; for older children/adolescents ask about any Internet sites of which their parents would not approve)

    f. Cultural context (migration history, ethnic identifications, religious affiliations, etc.)

    g. Trauma history (physical or sexual abuse, neglect, witnessing violence) and level of psychosocial adversity

    h. Substance use

    i. Legal history and risk-taking behaviors

    j. Sexual behavior

    k. Child and family strengths and weaknesses

6. Family history
   a. Family constellation/genogram
   b. Parental employment
   c. Psychiatric, learning, legal, substance abuse, or medical difficulties of genetically related family members
7. Mental status examination
   a. Appearance and behavior: grooming, dress, dysmorphia, injuries, eye contact
   b. Ability to cooperate/social relatedness
   c. Speech and language: fluency, volume, rate, and language skills
   d. Motor function: activity level, attention, impulsivity, coordination, tics
   e. Mood and affect: neurovegetative symptoms, manic symptoms, range of affect
   f. Thought process and content: psychotic symptoms (hallucinations, delusions, thought disorder)
   g. Anxiety: fears and phobias, obsessions or compulsions, posttraumatic anxiety
   h. Conduct symptoms: oppositionality, aggression (verbal or physical)
   i. History of trauma
   j. Assessment of risk: suicidal or self-abusive thoughts/behavior, thoughts or plans to harm others, sexual behaviors, Internet usage, legal issues, cigarettes, substance or alcohol usage
   k. Cognitive functioning: clinical estimate of cognitive skills and development
   l. Insight and judgment
8. Clinical formulation (including strengths and prognosis)
9. Diagnosis (DSM-IVTR)
10. Treatment recommendations

Psychiatric Review of Symptoms

Developmental delay:_____
Social relatedness:_____
Learning issues:_____
Enuresis/encopresis:_____
Tics:_____
Substance use:_____
Safety to self and others:_____

Depression
- Symptoms (5/9, 2 weeks): ___ depressed mood
  ___ sleep disorder ___ interest deficit ___ guilt
  ___ energy deficit ___ concentration deficit
  ___ appetite disorder ___ psychomotor retardation/agitation
  ___ suicidality

Mania
- Symptoms (3+ for 1 week or severe):
  ___ distractibility ___ indiscretion
  ___ grandiosity ___ flight of ideas
  ___ activity increase ___ sleep deficit
  ___ talkativeness

Psychosis/schizophrenia
- Symptoms (2/5, 1 month): ___ delusions
  ___ hallucinations ___ disorganized speech
  ___ disorganized/catatonic behavior
  ___ negative symptoms
- Prodrome/residual (1/2, 6 months):
  ___ negative symptoms
  ___ 2 positive symptoms

Anxiety
- Separation anxiety (3+ for 4 weeks):
  ___ distress/separated ___ worry/attachment figure
  ___ worry about separation ___ school refusal
  ___ fear of being alone ___ fear of sleeping away
  ___ nightmares ___ physical complaints
- GAD (3/6, 6 months): ___restless ___ fatigue
  ___ conscious ___ irritable ___ muscle tension
  ___ insomnia
- Panic (4/13, recurrence + 1 month of worry):
  ___ shortness of breath ___ faint ___ palpitations
  ___ trembling ___ sweating ___ choking ___ nauseous
  ___ depersonalization/derealization ___ numbness/tingling

___ chest pain ___ fear of dying ___ fear of losing sanity
___ chills/hot
- OCD: ___ obsessions ___ compulsions ___ interfere/time consuming (not conscious)
- PTSD (1 month):
Re-experience (1/5): ___ memories ___ dreams ___ flashbacks
___ distress/re-exposure ___ physiologic reactivity/re-exposure
Avoidance (3/7): ___ thoughts/feelings ___ activities/situations
___ amnesia ___ less interest ___ estrangement ___ restricted affect ___ thought of no future
Arousal (2/5): ___ sleep ___ irritability ___ consciousness
___ hypervigilant ___ startle
- Social phobia (3/3): ___ fear/social ___ exposure/panic
___ avoid/social

Attention deficit hyperactivity disorder
- Inattentive (6/9):
___ careless mistakes ___ attention difficulty
___ listening problem ___ loses things ___ fails to finish
___ organization problem ___ reluctant/mental effort
___ forgetful ___ easily distracted
- Hyperactive/impulsive (6/9):
___ restless/runs ___ unable to wait
___ not play quietly ____ on the go ___ fidgets
___ answers blurted ___ doesn't stay in seat
___ talks excessively ___ interrupts

Behavior disorder
- Oppositional defiant (4/8 last 6 months):
___ resentful ___ easily annoyed
___ argues/adults ___ loses temper
___ blames others ___ annoys deliberately
___ defies rules ___ spiteful
- Conduct disorder (3/15 past year + 1 past 6 months):
___ bullying ___ animal cruelty ___ destroying property
___ force sex ___ cruel ___ using weapon ___ set fires
___ break-ins ___ school refusal ___ everyday lying
___ stealing/confronting ___ stealing/not confronting
___ fighting ___ outlate ___ run away from home

Eating disorder
- Anorexia (4/4): ___ refuse/maintain weight
___ fear of fat ___ body distortion ___ amenorrhea
- Bulimia (5/5): ___ binge eating ___ lack/control
___ inappropriate weight/loss behavior
___ >2 times/week for 3 months
___ self-evaluation of body shape

Medication Appointment Record

Medication Appointment Record

Child's Name_____ D.O.B. _____ Date of Service _____

Current Medication: 1)_____ 3)_____

　　　　　　　　　　　2)_____ 4)_____

SUMMARY OF PROGRESS :_____
_____
_____
_____

CHANGES OF TARGET SYMPTOMS:

SYMPTOM	QUANTITATIVE INTENSITY AND FREQUENCY (CURRENT)

Current Physical Complaints: ☐No　　　☐Yes _____
Recent Injuries, Illnesses:　　　☐No　　☐Yes _____

Concurrent Medications:　　　　☐No　　☐Yes _____

Weight _____　　Height _____　　Blood pressure _____　Pulse _____

<u>SIDE EFFECTS:</u>

	Scale:	1–Mild	2–Moderate	3–Severe			
Side Effects	N	Y	Comment	**Side Effects**	N	Y	Comment
Fatigue, tiredness				Tremor			
Restlessness				Stiffness			
Increased activity				Slow movement			
Drowsiness				Poor coordination			
Difficulty sleeping				Poor memory			
Headache				Tics			
Dizziness				Other neurological			
Dry mouth				Constipation			
Blurred vision				Decreased appetite			
Hearing problems				Increased appetite			
Tinnitus				Weight gain			
Other ENT prob				Weight loss			
Difficulty breathing				Other GI symptoms			
Other respiratory prob				Difficulty urinating			
Palpitations				Enuresis			
Fainting				Other urinary symptom			
Other cardiovasc.Sx.				Itchiness			
Abdominal pain				Rashes			
Nausea				Sexual problems			
Vomiting				Other			
Diarrhea				Other			

MSE:_____
_____
_____

Changes in Diagnoses: _____
_____

GAF:

CLINICIAN-RATED GLOBAL IMPROVEMENT		
Rate total improvement, whether or not in your judgment it is due entirely to current treatment, compared to the patient's condition AT INITIAL EVALUATION. How much has patient changed?		
	0 – Not assessed	4 – Not changed
	1 – Very much improved	5 – Minimally worse
	2 – Much improved	6 – Much worse
	3 – Minimally improved	7 – Very much worse

Assessment/Plan_____
_____
_____
_____
_____

Medications Prescribed:
_____
_____

Next Appt _____ MD Name _____ Signature _____ Date _____

Abnormal Involuntary Movement Scale (AIMS)

Directions for administration: Ask patient to remove shoes and socks.

1. Ask patient to remove anything in his/her mouth.
2. Ask if there is anything wrong with his/her teeth. Dentures?
3. Ask patient if he/she notices any movements in mouth, face, hands, or feet. Ask if it bothers him/her or interferes with activities.
4. Have patient sit in firm, armless chair with both hands on knees, legs slightly apart, feet flat on floor. (Look at entire body for movements in this position.)
5. Ask patient to lean forward and let arms dangle. Look for movements.
6. Ask patient to open mouth. Observe for tongue movements. Repeat.
7. Ask patient to protrude tongue. Observe for tongue movements. Repeat.
8. Ask patient to tap thumb with each finger as rapidly as possible for 10–15 seconds first with right hand, then left. (Observe facial and leg movements.)
9. Flex and extend patient's right and left arms. (Note rigidity.)
10. Ask patient to stand up. (Observe body in profile.)
11. Ask patient to extend both arms outstretched in front with palms down. (Observe trunk, legs, and mouth.)
12. Have patient walk, turn, and come back. (Observe hands and gait.) Repeat.

RATINGS:

Facial and Oral Movements

1. Muscles of facial expression (e.g., movement of forehead, eyebrows, periorbital area, cheeks; include frowning, blinking, smiling, grimacing)
    None   1   2   3   4   5 Severe
2. Lips and perioral area (e.g,. puckering, pouting, smacking)
    None   1   2   3   4   5 Severe
3. Jaws (e.g., biting, clenching, chewing, mouth opening, lateral movement)
    None   1   2   3   4   5 Severe

4. Tongue (rate only increase in movement in and out of mouth)

> None   1   2   3   4   5 Severe

Extremity Movements

5. Upper (arms, wrist, hands, fingers). Include choreic movements (i.e., rapid, objectively purposeless, irregular, spontaneous), athetoid movements (i.e., slow, irregular, complex, serpentine). Do NOT include tremor.

> None   1   2   3   4   5 Severe

6. Lower (legs, knees, ankles, toes) (e.g., lateral knee movement, foot tapping, heel dropping, foot squirming, inversion and eversion of foot).

> None   1   2   3   4   5 Severe

Trunk Movements

7. Neck, shoulders, hips (e.g., rocking, twisting, squirming, pelvic gyrations)

> None   1   2   3   4   5 Severe

Global Judgments

8. Severity of abnormal movements:

> None   1   2   3   4   5 Severe

9. Incapacitation due to abnormal movements:

> None   1   2   3   4   5 Severe

10. Patient's awareness of abnormal movements:

> No awareness   1   2   3   4   5 Aware/Severe distress

11. Current problem with teeth (or dentures)?

> 1. No   2. Yes

12. Does patient wear dentures?

> 1. No   2. Yes

Test for tardive dyskinesia induced by antipsychotic medication.
Adapted from Department of Health and Human Services: Public Health Service; NIMH Treatment Strategies in Schizophrenia Study, ADM-117, 1985. (public domain)
http://www.mhsip.org/library/pdfFiles/abnormalinvoluntarymovementscale.pdf

The Simpson-Angus Scale (SAS)

1. Gait: Examine patient walking—his gait, swing of his arms, general posture.
   0. Normal
   1. Diminution of arm swing when walking
   2. Diminution of swing and rigidity in arms
   3. Stiff gait and arms held rigidly before the abdomen
   4. Shuffling gait with propulsion and retropulsion
2. Arm dropping: Patient and examiner raise arms to shoulder height and then let drop.
   0. Normal free fall with loud slap and rebound
   1. Fall slowed slightly—less audible slap and little rebound
   2. Fall slowed, no rebound
   3. Marked slowing; no slap
   4. Arms fall with resistance (as if through glue)
3. Shoulder shaking: Examiner bends arm at right angle, takes patient's left elbow in one hand, left hand in the other, and rotates arm and humerus. Repeats with right hand.
   0. Normal
   1. Slight stiffness and resistance
   2. Moderate stiffness and resistance
   3. Marked rigidity—difficulty with passive movement
   4. Extreme stiffness and almost frozen shoulder
4. Elbow rigidity: Passively bend and flex elbow while observing and palpating biceps.
   0. Normal
   1. Slight stiffness and resistance
   2. Moderate stiffness and rigidity
   3. Marked rigidity—difficult with passive movement
   4. Extreme stiffness and almost frozen elbow
5. Wrist rigidity: Examiner holds wrist in one hand and fingers in the other and passively bends and flexes wrist.
   0. Normal
   1. Slight stiffness and resistance
   2. Moderate stiffness and resistance
   3. Marked rigidity—difficulty with passive movement
   4. Extreme stiffness and almost frozen wrist
6. Leg pendulousness: Patient sits on exam table and legs swing freely. Examiner raises the leg and lets fall.
   0. Legs swing freely
   1. Slight diminution of leg swing

2. Moderate resistance to swing
3. Marked resistance and damping of swing
4. Complete absence of swing

7. Head dropping: Examiner has patient lie on exam table—lifts head up slightly and then drops.
   0. Head falls completely and quickly
   1. Slightly slowed fall of head and less thump
   2. Moderate slowing of head drop
   3. Head falls stiffly and slowly
   4. Head does not reach the examining table

8. Glabella tap: Patient told to open eyes wide and not blink. Glabella is tapped and number of successive blinks counted.
   0. 0–5 blinks
   1. 6–10 blinks
   2. 11–15 blinks
   3. 16–20 blinks
   4. 21+ blinks

9. Tremor: Patient observed walking normally.
   0. Normal
   1. Mild finger tremor
   2. Tremor of hand or arm occurring spasmodically
   3. Persistent tremor of one or more limbs
   4. Whole body tremor

10. Salivation: Patient is observed while talking and then asked to raise his tongue.
    0. Normal
    1. Excess salivation with some pooling
    2. Excess salivation and may interfere with talking
    3. Speaking with difficulty because of excess salivation
    4. Frank drooling

Test for extrapyramidal side effects of antipsychotic medication.
Adapted from Simpson GN, Angus JWS. A rating scale for extrapyramidal side effects. *Acta Psychiatr Scand* 1970;212(suppl 44):11–19.

Rating Scales

BROADBAND SCALES

Scale	Reporter	Age of Youth	Items	Supplier
Semistructured Diagnostic Scales				
Diagnostic Interview for Children (DISC 2.3)	Youth	9–17	Interview	a
	Parent	6–17	Interview	
Schizophrenia Affective Disorders (K-SADS)	Youth	9–17	Interview	b
	Parent	6–17	Interview	
Checklists				
Child Behavior Checklist (CBCL)				
Teacher Report Form (TRF)	Teacher/ parent	6–16	120	c
Caregiver Report Form (C-TRF)	Parent/ teacher	1.5–5	102	c
Youth Self-report (YSR)	Youth	11–18	105	c
Behavior Assessment Scale for Children (BASC-2)	Parent (preschool latency, adolesc)	2.0–18	134-160	d
	Teacher		139	d
	Youth self-report		65	d
Swanson, Nolan, Pelham-IV (SNAP-IV)	Parent or teacher	5–11	90	e
Brief Psychiatric Rating Scale for Children (BPRS-C)	Parent/ teacher	6–16	21	f

(a) DISC 2.3 Development Group, Columbia University: disc@childpsych.columbia.edu
(b) K-SADS, Western Psychiatric Institute and Clinic: www.wpic.pitt.edu/ksads
(c) ASEBA: www.aseba.org
(d) AGS Publishing: www.agsnet.com
(e) Swanson, Nolan, and Pelham-IV: www.adhd.net (public domain)
(f) *Psychopharmacol Bull* 1985;21(4):753–770. (public domain)

EXTERNALIZING DISORDERS

Scale	Reporter	Age of Youth	Items	Supplier
ADHD				
Conners Rating Scales, Revised (CRS-R)	Parent		80	a
	Teacher	3–18	59	a
	Youth self-report		87	a
Swanson, Nolan, Pelham-IV (SNAP-IV-Brief)	Parent or teacher	5–11	31	b
Behavioral Disorders				
Eyberg Child Behavior Inventory (ECBI)	Parent	2–16	36	c
Sutter-Eyberg Student Behavior Inventory (SESBI-R)	Teacher	2–16	38	c
Children's Aggression Scale	Parent	6–16	32	d
Overt Aggression Scale (OAS)	Parent	5–16	16	e
Young Mania Rating Scale (YMRS)	Clinician		11	f
	Adolescent	12–18	11	f
Nisonger Child Behavior Rating Form (CBRF)	Parent/teacher	5–15	66	g

(a) Connors rating scale: www.mhs.com

(b) Swanson, Nolan, and Pelham-IV: www.adhd.net (public domain)

(c) Eyberg SM, Pincus D: www.parinc.com

(d) Halperin JM, McKay KE, Newcorn JH. Development, reliability, and validity of the Children's Aggression Scale—Parent Version. *J Am Acad Child Adolesc Psychiatry* 2002;41(3):245–252.

(e) Yudofsky SC, Silver JM, Jackson W, Endicott J, Williams D. The overt aggression scale for the objective rating of verbal and physical aggression. *Am J Psychiatry* 1986;143(1):35–39.

(f) Young RC, Biggs JT, Ziegler VE, et al. A rating scale for mania: reliability, validity and sensitivity. *Br J Psychiatry* 1978;133:429–435.

(g) Aman MG, Tasse MJ, Rojahn J, Hammer D. The Nisonger CBRF: a child behavior rating form for children with developmental disabilities. *Research in Developmental Disabilities* 1996;17:41–57.

INTERNALIZING DISORDERS

Scale	Reporter	Age of Youth	Items	Supplier
Beck Depression Inventory (BDI)	Parent	3–18	80	a
	Teacher		59	a
	Youth self-report		87	a
Beck Hopelessness Scale	Youth self-report	11–18	20	a
Children's Depression Inventory (CDI)	Youth/parent/teacher	7–18	27	b
Center for Epidemiologic Studies—Depression Scale for Children (CES-DC)	Youth/parent	6–18	20	c
Children's Depression Rating Scale (CDRS-R)	Youth interview	6–12	60	d
Mood and Feelings Questionnaire (MFQ)	Parent/youth	11+	34	e
Screen for Child Anxiety and Related Emotional Disorders (SCARED)	Parent/youth	11+	41	f
Multidimensional Anxiety Scale for Children (MASC)	Youth/parent	6–18	39	b
Children's Manifest Anxiety Scale (CMAS-R)	Youth self-report	8–18	37	g
Social Phobia Anxiety Inventory for Children (SPAI-C)	Youth self-report	9–14	26	b

(a) BDI: www.psychcorp.com

(b) Multi-Health Systems: www.mhs.com

(c) Radloff LS. The CES-D Scale: a self-report depression scale for research in the general population. Applied Psychol Meas 1:385–401. (public domain, NIH, Epidemiology Branch)

(d) Poznanski EO, Freeman LN, Mokros HB. Children's depression rating scale—revised. Psychopharmacol Bull 1985;21(4):979–989. (public domain).

(e) Angold A and Costello EJ. Developmental Epidemiology Program, Duke University, 1987.

(f) Birmaher B, Khetarpal S, Brent D, et al. The Screen for Child Anxiety Related Emotional Disorders (SCARED): scale construction and psychometric characteristics. J Am Acad Child Adolesc Psychiatry 1997;36(4):545–553. (public domain)

(g) Reynolds CR, Richmond BO. Psychological Assessment Resources, Inc: www3.parinc.com, accessed July 2006.

SCALES ASSESSING OTHER DISORDERS

Scale	Reporter	Age of Youth	Items	Supplier
Eating Disorder				
SCOFF	Youth self-report	12–18	5	a
Obsessive-compulsive Disorder				
Yale-Brown Obsessive Compulsive Scale (Y-BOCS)	Clinician admin	6–18	69	b
Tic Disorders				
Yale Global Tic Severity Scale (YGTSS)	Clinician rated	all	5 scales	c
Autism				
Autism Diagnostic Observations Schedule Generic (ADOS-G)	Clinician rating of child	all	3 domains	d
Autism Diagnostic Interview (ADI-R)	Clinician interview of parent	all	3 domains	e
Schizophrenia				
Positive and Negative Syndrome Scale for Schizophrenia (PANSS)	Youth self-report	12–adult	30	f
Symptom Onset in Schizophrenia (SOS)	Self-/family	all	16	g
Substance Abuse Disorder				
Substance Abuse Subtle Screening Inventory (SASSI-A2)	Youth self-report	12–18	20	h
Personal Experience Screening Questionnaire (PESQ)	Youth self-report	12–18	40	i
Adolescent Diagnostic Interview (ADI)	Clinician interview	12–18	213	j
Trauma				
Trauma Symptom Checklist for Children (TSCC)	Clinician/parent	8 to 16 yr	22	k
Children's Post-Traumatic Stress-Reaction Index (CPTS-RI)	Clinician/Youth self-report	9–14	20	l

(Continued)

253

SCALES ASSESSING OTHER DISORDERS (continued)

Scale	Reporter	Age of Youth	Items	Supplier
Suicide Risk				
Child and Adolescent Suicide Potential Index (CASPI)	Youth self-report	9–18	36	m
Columbia Suicide Screen (CSS)	Youth self-report	12–18	8	n
Reasons for Living Inventory for Adolescents (RFL-A)	Youth self-report	12–18	12	o

(a) Morgan JF, Reid F, Lacey JH. The SCOFF questionnaire: assessment of a new screening tool for eating disorders. *BMJ* 1999;319:1467–1468. (public domain)

(b) Goodman WK, Price LH, Rasmussen SA, et al. The Yale-Brown Obsessive Compulsive Scale. *Arch Gen Psychiatry* 1989;46:1006–1011. (public domain)

(c) Leckman JF, Riddle MA, Hardin MT, Ort SI, et al. The Yale Global Tic Severity Scale: Initial testing of a clinician-rated scale of tic severity. *J Am Acad Child Adolesc Psychiatry* 1989;28:566–573.

(d) Lord C, Rutter M, Goode S, et al. Autism diagnostic observation schedule: a standardized observation of communicative and social behavior. *J Autism Dev Disord* 1989;19:185–212. www.wpspublish.com

(e) Lord C, Rutter M, LeCouteur A. Autism Diagnostic Interview-Revised: a revised version of a diagnostic interview for caregivers of individuals with possible pervasive developmental disorders. *J Autism Dev Disord* 1994;24:659–685. www.wpspublish.com

(f) Kay SR, Fiszbein A, Opler LA. The positive and negative syndrome scale (PANSS) for schizophrenia. *Schizophr Bull* 1987;13:261–276.

(g) Perkins DO, Leserman J, Jarskog LF, et al. Characterizing and dating the onset of symptoms in psychotic illness: the Symptom Onset in Schizophrenia (SOS) inventory. *Schizophr Res* 2000;44:1–10.

(h) www.sassi.com

(i) Winters K. *Manual for the Personal Experience Screening Questionnaire (PESQ)*. Los Angeles: Western Psychological Services, 1991.

(j) Winters K, Henly G. *Adolescent Diagnostic Interview (ADI) Manual*. Los Angeles: Western Psychological Services, 1993.

(l) Trauma Symptom Checklist—Psychological Assessment Resources: www.parinc.com

(l) Pynoos RS: rpynoos@npih.medsch.ucla.edu

(m) Pfeffer CR: cpfeffer@med.cornell.edu

(n) Shaffer D, Scott M, Wilcox MA: www.teenscreen.org

(o) Gutierrez PM, Osman A, Kopper BA, Barrios FX. Why young people do not kill themselves: the reasons for living inventory for adolescents. *J Clin Child Psychol* 2000;29:177–187.

254

SCALES ASSESSING FUNCTIONAL IMPAIRMENT

Scale	Reporter	Age of Youth	Items	Supplier
Vineland Adaptive Behavior Scale (VABS-II)	Clinical interview of parent	0–18	287	a
Columbia Impairment Scale (CIS)	Lay interview of parent	7–9	13	b
Children's Global Assessment Scale (CGAS)	Clinician	4–16	1	b
Child and Adolescent Functional Assessment Scale (CAFAS)	Clinician or parent interview	5–16	164	c
Clinical Global Impressions (CGI)	Clinician	any age	7	d

(a) Sparrow SS, Cicchetti DV, Balla DA: www.agsnet.com
(b) Bird HR. The assessment of functional impairment. In: Shaffer D, Lucas CP, Richters JE, eds. *Diagnostic assessment in child and adolescent psychopathology.* New York: Guilford Press, 209–229. (public domain)
(c) Hodges K. Functional Assessment Systems: www.cafas.com
(d) CGI. *Psychopharm Bull* 1985;21(4):839. (public domain)

SCALES ASSESSING FAMILY FUNCTIONING

Scale	Reporter	Age of Youth	Items	Supplier
Family Environment Scale (FES)	Parent/youth	11–adult	90	a
Caregiver Strain Questionnaire (CSQ)	Parent	all ages	21	b
Family Adaptability and Cohesion Evaluation Scale (FACES-III)	Clinician	families	3 scales	c
Family Assessment Devise (FAD)	Self	all	60	d
Family Assessment Measure	Youth/adult	10 to adult	50	e
Parenting Stress Index	Parent	0–12	101	e
Parenting Satisfaction Scale	Parent	6–14	45	f

(a) Moos BS, Moos RH; MindGarden: info@mindgarden.com

(b) Brannan AM, Heflinger CA, and Bickman L. The Caregiver Strain Questionnaire: measuring the impact on the family of living with a child with serious emotional problems. *J Emotional Behavioral Disorders* 1997;5(4):212–223.

(c) Olson DH. Circumplex Model VII: Validation studies and FACES III. *Family Process* 1986;25:337–351.

(d) Miller IW, Epstein NB, Baldwin LM. The McMaster Family Assessment Device. *J Marital Family Therapy* 1985;1(4):345–356.

(e) Psychological Assessment Resources: www.parinc.com, accessed July 2006.

(f) PsychCorp: www.harcourtassessment.com, accessed July 2006.

Commonly Used Tests: Assessment of Children and Youth

Test	Test Age Range	Supplier
Intelligence		
Stanford-Binet	2–23 yr	a
WPPSI-III	2:6–7:3 yr	b
WISC-IV	6–16:11 yr	b
WASI	6–89 yr	b
K-ABC-II	2:5–2:5 yr	c
Leiter	all ages	c
TONI	6–85 yr	c
Achievement		
KTEA	4:6–90 yr	d
WIAT	4–85 yr	b
Wide Range Achievement Test	5–85 yr	b, c
Adaptive		
AAMR	3–21 yr	c
Adaptive Behavior Assessment System-II	0–89 yr	d
Vineland Adaptive Behavior Scales-II	0–18:11 yr	d
Personality Self-Report		
Jesness Inventory Revised	8 yr and older	f
MMPI	14 yr and older	g
Personality Inventory For Youth	9–19 yr	b, c
Million Adolescent Clinical Inventory	13–19 yr	g
Projective		
Rorschach	5 yr and older	b, c, g
Thematic Apperception Test	4 yr and older	b, c, g
Neuropsychological		
NEPSY	3–12 yr	b, c
WRAML 2	5–90 yr	b, c

Test	Test Age Range	Supplier
Memory		
Rey-Osterrieth Complex Figure Test	5–94 yr	c
Wisconsin Card Sorting Test	6.5–89 yr	c

WPPSI, Wechsler Preschool and Primary Scale of Intelligence; WISC, Wechsler Intelligence Scale for Children; WASI, Wechsler Abbreviated Scale of Intelligence; K-ABC-II, Kaufman Assessment Battery for Children, second edition; Test of Nonverbal Intelligence (TONI); KTEA, Kaufman Test of Educational Achievement; WIAT, Wechsler Individual Achievement Test II; AAMR, Adaptive Behavior Scale; BASC-2, Behavior Assessment System for Children, second edition; MMPI, Minnesota Multiphasic Personality Inventory; NEPSY, A Developmental Neuropsychological Assessment; WRAML 2, Wide Range Assessment of Memory and Learning, second edition.

Suppliers:
(a) Riverside Publishing Company, www.riverpub.com
(b) PsychCorp, www.harcourtassessment.com
(c) Psychological Assessment Resources, www.parinc.com
(d) AGS Publishing, www.agsnet.com
(e) ASEBA Research Center, www.ASEBA.org
(f) Multi Health Systems, www.mhs.com
(g) Pearson Assessments, www.pearsonassessments.com

ADHD: Inattentive	**CALL FOR FrEd** (6/9)
Hyperactive-Impulsive	**RUNS FASTT** (6/9)
Oppositional defiant disorder	**REAL BADS** (4/8)
Conduct disorder	**BAD FOR A BUSINESS** (3/15 past yr; 1 past mo)
Separation anxiety	**PUSH NAGS** (3/8)
PTSD	**R**emembers (1) **A**trocious (3) **A**ttacks (2)
Major depression	**SIG E CAPS** (4/8)
Manic episode	**DIGFAST** (3/7)
Schizophrenia	**D**elusions **H**erald **S**chizophrenic's **B**ad **N**ews (2/5)
Anorexia nervosa	**W**eight **F**ear **B**others **A**norexics (4/4)
Bulimia nervosa	**B**ulimics **O**ver-**C**onsume **P**astries (4/4)
Substance abuse	**T**empted **W**ith **C**ognac (3/7)
Alcoholism	**CAGE** (2/4)

4   Resources for Parents

General
American Academy of Child and Adolescent Psychiatry
Facts for Families
www.aacap.org

American Academy of Pediatrics
www.aap.org

National Alliance for the Mentally Ill (NAMI)
www.nami.org

Medication
Dulcan MK, Lizarralde C. *Helping parents, youth, and teachers understand medications for behavioral and emotional problems. A resource book of medication information handouts. 2nd ed.* Washington, DC: American Psychiatric Publishing, 2003.

Wilens TE. *Straight talk about psychiatric medications for kids.* New York: Guilford Press, 1999.

Anxiety Disorders
DuPont Spencer E, Dupont R, Dupont C. *The anxiety cure for kids: a guide for parents.* Hoboken, NJ: John Wiley & Sons, 2003.

Attention Deficit Hyperactivity Disorder
Barkley RA. *Taking charge of ADHD: the complete authoritative guide for parents.* New York: Guilford Press, 1995.
Children and Adults with Attention Deficit Hyperactivity Disorder (CHADD). http://www.chadd.org
National Attention Deficit Disorder Association (ADDA). http://www.add.org

Autism
Autism Society of America. http://www.autism-society.org
Siegel B. *Help children with autism learn: a guide to treatment approaches for parents and teachers.* Oxford: Oxford University Press, 2003.

Eating Disorders
Marcontell D, Michel SG, Willard A. *When dieting becomes dangerous: a guide to understanding and treating anorexia and bulimia.* New Haven: Yale University Press, 2003.

Learning Disabilities
National Center for Learning Disabilities. www.ncld.org

Mood Disorders
Fristad MA, Goldberg Arnold JS. *Raising a moody child: how to cope with depression and bipolar disorder.* New York: Guilford Press, 2004.

Miklowitz DJ. *The bipolar disorder survival guide: what you and your family need to know.* New York: Guilford Press, 2002.

Papolos DE, Papolos J. *The bipolar child: the definitive and reassuring guide to childhood's most misunderstood disorder.* New York: Broadway Books, 2002.

The Depression and Bipolar Support Alliance. www.dbsalliance.org

Bipolar Disorders Information Center. http://mhsorce.com/bipolar/

Obsessive Compulsive Disorder
Chansky T. *Freeing your child from obsessive-compulsive disorder: a powerful, practical program for parents of children and adolescents.* New York: Three Rivers Press, 2001.

Obsessive-Compulsive Foundation. http://www.familymanagement.com/facts

Substance Abuse
Schaefer D, Espeland P., eds. *Choices and consequences: what to do when a teenager uses drugs/alcohol: a step-by-step system that really works.* New York: New American Library Trade, 1998

Tourette Syndrome
Haerle T, Eisnreich J. *Children with Tourette Syndrome: a parent's guide (special needs collection).* Bethesda, MD: Woodbine House, 2003.

Tourette Syndrome Association. www.tsa-usa.org

Suggested Readings

Abelson JF, Kwan KY, O'Roak BJ, et al. Sequence variants in *SLITRK1* are associated with Tourette's Syndrome. *Science* 2005;October 14:317–320.

Amaya-Jackson L, Reynold V, Murray MC, et al. Cognitive-behavioral treatment for pediatric posttraumatic stress disorder: protocol and application in school and community settings. *Cogn Behav Practice* 2003;10(3):204–213.

American Academy of Child and Adolescent Psychiatry. Practice parameters for the psychiatric assessment of children and adolescents. *J Am Acad Child Adolesc Psychiatry* 1997;36(10 Suppl):4S–20S.

American Academy of Child and Adolescent Psychiatry. Practice parameters for the psychiatric assessment and treatment of children and adolescents with bipolar disorder. *J Am Acad Child Adolesc Psychiatry* 1997;36:138–157.

American Academy of Child and Adolescent Psychiatry. Practice parameters for the assessment and treatment of children and adolescents with schizophrenia. *J Am Acad Child Adolesc Psychiatry* 2001;40(Suppl):4S–23S.

American Academy of Child and Adolescent Psychiatry. Practice parameters for the assessment and treatment of children and adolescents with suicidal behavior. *J Am Acad Child Adolesc Psychiatry* 2001;40(7 Suppl):24S–51S.

American Academy of Child and Adolescent Psychiatry. Practice parameters for the assessment and treatment of children and adolescents with reactive attachment disorder of infancy and early childhood. *J Am Acad Child Adolesc Psychiatry* 2005;44:1206–1219.

American Academy of Child and Adolescent Psychiatry (AACAP). Committee on Mental Retardation and Developmental Disabilities: The roles and responsibilities of child and adolescent psychiatry in the field of developmental disabilities. *Am Acad Child Adolesc Psychiatry News,* Winter 1988;7.

American Academy of Pediatrics, Committee on Child Abuse and Neglect. Guidelines for the evaluation of sexual abuse of children. *Pediatrics* 1991;87:254–260.

American Psychiatric Association. *Diagnostic and Statistical Manual of Mental Disorders.* 4th ed. (text rev.). Washington, DC: American Psychiatric Association, 2000.

American Psychological Association, Task Force on Promotion and Dissemination of Psychological Procedures. Training in and dissemination of empirically validated psychological treatments. *Clin Psychologist* 1995;48:3–23.

Asarnow JR, Carlson GA. Childhood depression: five-year outcome following combined cognitive behavioral therapy and pharmacotherapy. *Am J Psychother* 1988;42:456–464.

Barkley RA. Psychosocial treatments for attention-deficit hyperactivity disorder in children. *J Clin Psychiatry* 2002;63(Suppl. 12): 36–43.

Barret PM, Duffy AL, Dadds MR, et al. Cognitive-behavioral treatment of anxiety disorders in children: long-term (6-year) follow-up. *J Consult Clin Psychol* 2001;69:135–141.

Beidel DC, Turner SM, Hamlin K, et al. The Social Phobia and Anxiety Inventory for Children (SPAI-C): external and discriminative validity. *Behav Ther* 2000;31:75–87.

Bernstein GA, Layne AE, Egan EA, et al. School-based intervention for anxious children. *J Am Acad Child Adolesc Psychiatry* 2005;44: 1118–1127.

Birmaher B, Khetarpal S, Brent D, et al. The Screen for Child Anxiety Related Emotional Disorders (SCARED): scale construction and psychometric characteristics. *J Am Acad Child Adolesc Psychiatry* 1997;36:545–553.

Birmaher B, Ryan ND, Williamson DE, et al. Childhood and adolescent depression: a review of the past 10 years. Part I. *J Am Acad Child Adolesc Psychiatry* 1996;35(11):1427–1439.

Bloch MH, Peterson BS, Scahill L, et al. Adulthood outcome of tic and obsessive-compulsive symptom severity in children with Tourette syndrome. *Arch Pediatr Adolesc Med* 2006;160(1):65–69.

Bolton P, MacDonald H, Pickles A, et al. A case-control family history study of autism. *J Child Psychol Psychiatry* 1994;35:877–900.

Brent DA, Holder D, Kolko D, et al. A clinical psychotherapy trial for adolescent depression comparing cognitive, supportive, and family therapy. *Arch Gen Psychiatry* 1997;54:877–885.

Briere J, Johnson K, Bissada A, et al. The Trauma Symptom Checklist for Young Children: reliability and association with abuse exposure in a multisite study. *Child Abuse Negl* 2001;25:1001–1014.

Burack JS, Hodapp RM, and Zigler E, eds. *Handbook of Mental Retardation and Development.* New York: Cambridge University Press, 1998.

Carlson GA, Kashani JH. Manic symptoms in a non-referred adolescent population. *J Affect Disord* 1988;15:219–226.

Carlat DJ. *The Psychiatric Interview.* 2nd ed. Practical Guides in Psychiatry. Philadelphia: Lippincott Williams & Wilkins, 2005.

Cheng K, Myers KM. *Child and Adolescent Psychiatry: The Essentials.* Philadelphia: Lippincott Williams & Wilkins, 2005.

ChildStats (*http://www.childstats.gov*). National Center for Children Exposed to Violence (*http://www.nccev.org*).

Clarke GN, Rohde P, Lewinsohn PM, et al. Cognitive behavioral group treatment of adolescent depression: efficacy of acute treatment and booster sessions. *J Am Acad Child Adolesc Psychiatry* 1999;38:272–279.

Cohen JA. Practice parameters for the assessment and treatment of children and adolescents with posttraumatic stress disorder. *J Am Acad Child Adolesc Psychiatry* 1998;37(10, Suppl):4S–26S.

Cohen JA, Deblinger E, Mannarino AP, et al. A multisite, randomized controlled trial for children with sexual abuse-related PTSD symptoms. *J Am Acad Child Adolesc Psychiatry* 2004;43:393–402.

Connor DF, Meltzer BM. *Pediatric Psychopharmacology: Fast Facts*. New York: W.W. Norton & Co., 2006.

Costello EJ, Mustillo S, Erkanli A, et al. Prevalence and development of psychiatric disorder in childhood and adolescence. *Arch Gen Psychiatry* 2003;60:837–844.

Costello EJ, Pine DS, Hammen C, et al. Development and natural history of mood disorders: advances. *Child Adolesc Psychiatr Clin N Am* 2000; 9:159–182.

DeBellis MD, Hall J, Boring AM, et al. A pilot longitudinal study of hippocampal volumes in pediatric maltreatment-related posttraumatic stress disorder. *Biol Psychiatry* 2001;50:305–309.

DeBettencourt LU. Understanding the differences between IDEA and Section 504. *Teaching Exceptional Children* 2002;34:16–23.

DeVeaugh-Geiss J, March J, Shapiro M, et al Child and adolescent psychopharmacology in the new millennium: a workshop for academia, industry, and government. *J Am Acad Child Adolesc Psychiatry* 2006;45:261–270.

Donnelly CL, Amaya-Jackson L, March JS. Psychopharmacology of pediatric posttraumatic stress disorder. *J Child Adolesc Psychopharmacol* 1999;9:203–220.

Dow SP, Sonies BC, Scheib D, et al. Practical guidelines for the assessment and treatment of selective mutism. *J Am Acad Child Adolesc Psychiatry* 1998;37:903–904.

Dulcan MK, Lizarralde C, eds. *Helping Parents, Youth, and Teachers Understand Medications for Behavioral and Emotional Problems: A Resource Book of Medication Information Handouts*. 2nd ed. Washington, DC: American Psychiatric Publishing, Inc., 2002.

Dulcan MK, Wiener JM, eds. *Essentials of Child and Adolescent Psychiatry*. Washington, DC: American Psychiatric Publishing, Inc., 2006.

Dykens EM. Annotation: psychopathology in children with intellectual disability. *J Child Psychol, Psychiatry* 2000;41:407–417.

Everly G, Mitchell JT. *Critical Incident Stress Management (CISM). A New Era and Standard of Care in Crisis Intervention*. Ellicott City, MD: Chevron Publishing, 1997.

Falloon IRH. Psychotherapy for schizophrenic disorders; a review. *Br J Hosp Med* 1992;48:164–170.

Feindler EL, Ecton RB, Kingley D, et al. Group anger-control training for institutionalized psychiatric male adolescents. *Behav Ther* 1986;17:109–123.

Geller B, DelBello MP, eds. *Bipolar Disorder in Childhood and Early Adolescence.* New York: Guilford Press, 2003.

Gray CA, Garand JD. Social stories: improving responses of students with autism with accurate social information. *Focus Autistic Behav* 1993;8:1–10.

Green WH. *Child and Adolescent Clinical Psychopharmacology.* New York: Lippincott Williams & Wilkins, 2001.

Greenspan S, Wieder S. Developmental patterns and outcomes in infants and children with disorder of relating and communicating: a chart review of 200 cases of children with autistic spectrum diagnoses. *J Dev Learn Dis* 1997;1:87–141.

Grice DE, Halmi KA, Fichter MM, et al. Evidence for a susceptibility gene for anorexia nervosa on chromosome 1. *Am J Hum Genet* 2002;70:787–792.

Grigsby RK. Mental health consultation at a youth shelter: An ethnographic approach. *Child Youth Care Forum* 1993;21:247–261.

Grindle CF, Remington B. Discrete-trial training for autistic children when reward is delayed: A comparison of conditioned cue value and response marking. *J Appl Behav Anal* 2002;35:187–190.

Group for Advancement of Psychiatry (GAP) Committee on Child Psychiatry. *The Process of Child Therapy.* New York: Brunner/Mazel, 1982.

Gutierrez PM, Osman A, Kopper BA, et al. Why young people do not kill themselves: The reasons for living inventory for adolescents. *J Clin Child Psychol* 2000;29:177–187.

Hall D, Leichner P, Calderon R, eds. *Meal Support Introduction for Parents, Friends, and Caregivers. Instruction Manual.* Seattle, WA: Children's Hospital and Regional Medical Center, 2004.

Halmi KA. Rating scales in the eating disorders. *Psychopharmacol Bull* 1985;21:1001–1043.

Harrison PJ, Owen MJ. Genes for schizophrenia? Recent findings and their pathophysiological implications. *Lancet* 2003;361:417–419.

Henggeler SW, Cunningham PB, Pickrel SG, et al. Multisystemic therapy: an effective violence prevention approach for serious juvenile offenders. *J Adolesc* 1996;19:47–61.

Herman S. Practice parameters for child custody evaluations. *J Am Acad Child Adolesc Psychiatry* 1997;36:575–685.

Hood KK, Eyberg SM. Outcomes of parent-child interaction therapy: mother's reports of maintenance three to six years after treatment. *J Clin Child Adolesc Psychol* 2003;32:419–429.

Hughes CW, Emslie GJ, Crimson ML, et al. The Texas children's medication algorithm project: report of the Texas consensus conference panel on medication treatment of childhood major depressive disorder. *J Am Acad Child Adolesc Psychiatry* 1999;38(11):1442–1454.

Jacobsen JK, Giedd JN, Castellanos FX, et al. Progressive reduction of temporal lobe structures in childhood-onset schizophrenia. *Am J Psychiatry* 1998;155:678–685.

Johnson LD, O'Malley PM, Bachman JG, et al. Monitoring the Future National Results on Adolescent Drug Use: Overview of Key Findings, 2003. Bethesda, MD: NIDA, NIH Publication No. 03-5374, 2004.

Kaminer Y, Jellinek S. Contingency management reinforcement procedures for adolescent substance abuse. *J Am Acad Child Adolesc Psychiatry* 2000;39:1324–1326.

Katz LY, Cox BJ, Gunasekara S, et al. Feasibility of dialectic behavior therapy for suicidal adolescent inpatients. *J Am Acad Child Adolesc Psychiatry* 2004;43:276–282.

Kay SR, Opler, LA, Lindenmayer JP, et al. Reliability and validity of the positive and negative syndrome scale for schizophrenics. *Psychiatry Res* 1988:23;99–110.

Kazdin A, Weiss J, eds. *Evidence-based Psychotherapies for Children and Adolescents.* New York: Guilford Press, 2003.

Kinoy BP. *Eating Disorders: New Directions in Treatment and Recovery.* New York: Columbia University Press, 2001.

Koplewicz H. *More Than Moody: Recognizing and Treating Adolescent Depression.* New York: G.P. Putnam's Sons, 2002.

Last CG, Hersen M, Kazdin AD, et al. Comparison of DSM-III separation anxiety and overanxious disorders: demographic characteristics and patterns of comorbidity. *J Am Acad Child Adolesc Psychiatry* 1987;26:527–531.

Lewis DO, Yeager CA, eds. Juvenile violence. *Child Adolesc Psychiatr Clin N Am* 2000;9:733–891.

Lieberman JA, Stroup TS, McEvoy JP, et al. (Clinical Antipsychotic Trials of Intervention Effectiveness [CATIE] Investigators). Effectiveness of antipsychotic drugs in patients with chronic schizophrenia. *N Engl J Med* 2005;353:1209–1223.

Linehan MM, Heard HL, Armstrong HE. Naturalistic follow-up of a behavioral treatment for chronically parasuicidal borderline patients. *Arch Gen Psychiatry* 1993;50:971–974.

Lochman JE, Nelson WM, Sims JP. A cognitive-behavioral program for use with aggressive children. *Clin Child Psychol* 1981;10:146–148.

Lovaas OI. Behavioral treatment and normal educational and intellectual functioning in young autistic children. *Consult Clin Psychol* 1987;55:3–9.

Madigan A, Dowell K. *Emerging Practices in the Prevention of Child Abuse and Neglect.* Washington, DC: U.S. Department of Health and Human Services, 2003.

Marans S, Cohen D. Children and inner-city violence: strategies for intervention. In: Leavitt L, Fox N, eds. *Psychological Effects of War and Violence on Children.* Hillsdale, NJ: LEA, 1993:281–301.

March JS, Franklin M, Nelson A, et al. Cognitive-behavioral psychotherapy for pediatric obsessive-compulsive disorder. *J Clin Child Psychol* 2001;30:8–18.

March JS, Leonard HL. Obsessive-compulsive disorder in children and adolescents: a review of the past 10 years. *J Am Acad Child Adolesc Psychiatry* 1996;35:1265–1273.

Martin A, Scahill L, Charney DS, Leckman JF, eds. *Pediatric Psychopharmacology.* New York: Oxford University Press, 2003.

Mikkelson EJ. Enuresis and encopresis: ten years of progress. *J Am Acad Child Adolesc Psychiatry* 2001;40:1146–1158.

Miller GA. *The Substance Abuse Subtle Screening Inventory (SASSI): Manual.* 2nd ed. Springfield, IN: The SASSI Institute, 1999.

Miller I, Kabacoff R, Epstein N. Development of a clinical rating scale for the McMaster model of family functioning. *Family Process* 1994;33:53–69.

Mitchell JT, Everly GS. *Critical Incident Stress Debriefing: An Operations Manual.* Ellicott City, MD: Chevron, 1996.

Moos R, Moos B. *Family Environment Scale Manual.* Palo Alto, CA: Consulting Psychologists Press, 1980.

Morgan JF, Reid F, Lacey JH. The SCOFF questionnaire: assessment of a new screening tool for eating disorders. *BMJ* 1999;319:1467–1468.

Mufson L, Weissman MM, Moreau D, et al. Efficacy of interpersonal psychotherapy for depressed adolescents. *Arch Gen Psychiatry* 1999;56:573–579.

National Institutes of Health (NIH). Tourette Syndrome Fact Sheet (*http://www.ninds.nih.gov/disorders/tourette/detail_tourette.htm*)

Newcorn JH, Strain J. Adjustment disorder in children and adolescents. *J Am Acad Child Adolesc Psychiatry* 1992;31:318–326.

Ollendick TH, March J, eds. *Phobic and Anxiety Disorders in Children and Adolescents: A Clinician's Guide to Effective Psychosocial and Pharmacological Interventions.* New York: Oxford University Press, 2003.

Olson DH, McCubbin HI, Barnes H. *FACES III: Family Adaptability and Cohesion Evaluation Scales.* St. Paul, MN: University of Minnesota, Family Social Science, 1982.

Osterling J, Dawson G, Munson J. Early recognition of 1-year-old infants with autism spectrum disorder versus mental retardation. *Dev Psychopathol* 2002;14:239–251.

Patterson GR, Ray RS, Shaw DA. Direct intervention in families of deviant children. *Oregon Res Inst Res Bull* 1968;8:1–11.

Pavuluri MN, Birmaher B, Naylor MW. Pediatric bipolar disorder: a review of the past 10 years. *J Am Acad Child Adolesc Psychiatry* 2005;44:846–871.

Pelham WE, Gnagy EM, Greiner AR, et al. Behavioral versus behavioral and pharmacological treatment in ADHD children attending a summer treatment program. *J Abnorm Child Psychol* 2000; 28:507–525.

Pruett K, Pruett M. Only God decides: young children's perception of divorce and the legal system. *J Am Acad Child Adolesc Psychiatry* 1999;38:12.

Roberts R, Mather N. Legal protections for individuals with learning disabilities: The IDEA, Section 504, and the ADA. *Learn Disabilities Res Practice* 1995;10:160–168.

Rosenwasser B, Axelrod S. The contribution of applied behavior analysis to the education of people with autism. *Behav Modif* 2001;25:671–677.

Scahill L, Riddle M, McSwiggen-Hardin M, et al. Children's Yale-Brown obsessive compulsive scale: reliability and validity. *J Am Acad Child Adolesc Psychiatry* 1997;36:844–852.

Stahl SM, Stahl SM, Grady MM, eds. *Essential Psychopharmacology: The Prescriber's Guide.* Cambridge, UK: Cambridge University Press, 2004.

Steiner H, Cauffman E. Juvenile justice, delinquency, and psychiatry. *Child Adolesc Psychiatr Clin N Am* 1998;7:653–672.

Perkins DO, Leserman J, Jarskog LF, et al. Characterizing and dating the onset of symptoms in psychotic illness: The Symptom Onset in Schizophrenia (SOS) inventory. *Schizophrenia Res* 2000:44;1–10.

Pfeffer C, ed. *Severe Stress and Mental Disturbance in Children.* Washington, DC: American Psychiatric Press, 1996.

Pfeffer CR, Jiang H, Kakuma T. Child-Adolescent Suicidal Potential Index (CASPI): a screen for risk for early onset suicidal behavior. *Psychol Assess* 2000;12:304–318.

Schetky DH, Benedek EP, eds. *Principles and Practice of Child and Adolescent Forensic Psychiatry.* Washington, DC: American Psychiatric Publishing Inc., 2002:191–203.

Schopler E. Implementation of the TEACCH philosophy. In: Cohen DJ, Volkmar FR, eds. *Handbook of Autism and Pervasive Developmental Disorders.* 2nd ed. New York: Wiley, 1997:767–795.

Schwab-Stone ME, Ayers TS, Kasprow W. No safe haven: a study of violence exposure in an urban community. *J Am Acad Child Adolesc Psychiatry* 1995;34:1451–1459.

Shaffer D, Greenberg T. Suicide and suicidal behavior in children and adolescents. In: Shaffer D, Waslick BD, eds. *The Many Faces of Depression in Children and Adolescents.* Washington, DC: American Psychiatric Publishing Inc., 2002:129–178.

Shaffer D, Scott M, Wilcox H, et al. The Columbia Suicide Screen: validity and reliability of a screen for youth suicide and depression. *J Am Acad Child Adolesc Psychiatry* 2004;43:71–79.

Sloboda Z, David SL. *Preventing Drug Use among Children and Adolescents: A Research Based Guide.* Bethesda, MD: NIDA, NIH, Publication No. 04-4212A, 2003.

Sparrow SS, Cicchetti DV, Balla DA. *Vineland Adaptive Behavior Scales.* 2nd ed. Circle Pines, MN: AGS Publishing, 2005.

State MW, Lombroso PH, Pauls DL, et al. The genetics of childhood psychiatric disorders: a decade of progress. *J Am Acad Child Adolesc Psychiatry* 2000;39:946–962.

Steiner H, Lock J. Anorexia nervosa and bulimia nervosa in children and adolescents: a review of the past 10 years. *J Am Acad Child Adolesc Psychiatry* 1998;37:352–359.

Stice E, Telch CF, Rizvi SL. Development and validation of the eating disorder diagnostic scale. *Development* 2000;12:123–131.

Still GF. The Coulston lectures on some abnormal physical conditions in children. *Lancet* 1902;1:1008–1012.

Strober M. Managing the chronic, treatment-resistant patient with anorexia nervosa. *Int J Eat Disord* 2004;36:245–255.

Stubbe DE, ed. *Attention-deficit/Hyperactivity Disorder.* Child and Adolescent Psychiatric Clinics of North America, vol. 9. Philadelphia: WB Saunders, 2000.

Swedo, SE, Leonard HL, Garvey M, et al. Pediatric autoimmune neuropsychiatric disorders associated with streptococcal infections (PANDAS): clinical description of the first fifty cases. *Am J Psychiatry* 1998;155:264–271.

Terr L. *Too Scared to Cry: Psychic Trauma in Childhood.* New York: Basic Books, 1992.

Tourette's Syndrome Study Group. Treatment of ADHD in children with tics: a randomized controlled trial. *Neurology* 2002;58(4): 527–536.

Treatment for Adolescents With Depression Study Team. Fluoxetine, cognitive-behavioral therapy, and their combination for adolescents with depression: Treatment for Adolescents With Depression Study (TADS) randomized controlled trial. *JAMA* 2004;292: 807–820.

Vitiello B, Stoff DM. Subtypes of aggression and their relevance to child psychiatry. *J Am Acad Child Psychiatry* 1997;36:307–315.

Webster-Stratton C, Hammond M. Treating children with early-onset conduct problems: a comparison of parent and child training interventions. *J Consul Clin Psychol* 1997;65:93–109.

Weisz JR, Thurber CA, Sweeney L, et al. Brief treatment of mild to moderate child depression using primary and secondary control enhancement training. *J Consult Clin Psychol* 1997;65:703–707.

Whelan E, Cooper PJ. The association between childhood feeding problems and maternal eating disorder: a community study. *Psychol Med* 2000;30:69–77.

Wilens TE. Does stimulant therapy of attention-deficit/hyperactivity disorder beget later substance abuse? A meta-analytic review of the literature. *Pediatrics* 2003;111:179–185.

Woolston JL. Theoretical considerations of the adjustment disorders. *J Am Acad Child Adolesc Psychiatry* 1988;27:280–287.

Yehuda R, ed. *Treating Trauma Survivors with PTSD*. Washington, DC: American Psychiatric Publishing Inc., 2002.

Youngstrom EA, Findling RL, Calabrese JR, et al. Comparing the diagnostic accuracy of six potential screening instruments for bipolar disorder in youth aged 5 to 17 years. *J Am Acad Child Adolesc Psychiatry* 2004;43:847–858.

Yudofsky SC, Silver JM, Jackson W, et al. The overt aggression scale for the objective rating of verbal and physical aggression. *Am J Psychiatry* 1986;143:35–39.

Index

Note: Page numbers followed by *f, b,* or *t* refer to figures, boxes, and tables, respectively.